Madam Politician

MADAM POLITICIAN

The Women at the Table of
Irish Political Power

MARTINA FITZGERALD

Gill Books

Gill Books
Hume Avenue
Park West
Dublin 12
www.gillbooks.ie

Gill Books is an imprint of M.H. Gill & Co.

978 07171 8143 8

Print origination by O'K Graphic Design, Dublin
Copy-edited by Ruth Mahony
Proofread by Djinn von Noorden
Printed by CPI Group (UK) Ltd, Croydon CRO 4YY

This book is typeset in 11/16 pt Minion.

The paper used in this book comes from the wood pulp of managed forests.
For every tree felled, at least one tree is planted, thereby renewing natural
resources.

A CIP catalogue record for this book is available from the British Library.

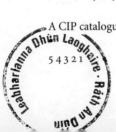

5 4 3 2 1

Acknowledgements

Countess Constance Markievicz, the first Irish woman to be appointed a senior government minister, often shed her title and favoured being called by the more democratic 'Madame'. In the pre-Independence era in Ireland, many nationalist women abandoned the English-used titles of 'Mrs' and 'Ms' and – in the French republican tradition – styled themselves as 'Madame'.[1]

Today, female cabinet members in the United States are well used to being addressed as 'Madam Secretary'. As yet, the title 'Madam President' has only featured in movies and in television programmes. At Westminster, the first female Speaker of the House of Commons, Betty Boothroyd, was addressed as 'Madam Speaker'. Considering these associations, it is highly appropriate that my book based on the experiences of Ireland's two former female presidents and the seventeen surviving women who have served as senior government ministers should be titled *Madam Politician*.

I could not have written this book without the co-operation of these remarkable women, all of whom readily agreed to my requests for interviews and gave generously of their time in meeting with me. Only two women have been elected president of Ireland and only nineteen women have served as senior cabinet ministers. All but two of these women (Markievicz and Eileen Desmond) are alive today. *Madam Politician* draws on my interviews with these nineteen women. In their words and recollections, their voices are collectively heard for the first time on getting onto the ladder in Irish politics and climbing to the top.

My book has political settings – Leinster House, Government Buildings and Áras an Uachtaráin – but its themes are universal. Many will empathise with these women who remain a rare species in their workplace and who have battled to have their voices heard and counted while balancing a career with family life. As public figures, they have also had to deal with an enduring focus on appearance and sexism in political life. *Madam Politician* is set in the political sphere, but it really encapsulates the challenges and triumphs – and the disappointments and despairs – of all women in a changing Irish society.

In writing this book, I owe thanks to many friends and colleagues including Kevin Rafter, Geoffrey Shannon, Ailbhe Conneely, Sorcha Ní Riada, Treasa O'Sullivan, Charlotte Brenner, Sile O'Neill, Stephen McKenna, Eimear Keogan, Helen Kelleher, Michelle Browne and Kate Egan. Many thanks also to Valerie Cox, Karl Deeter, Patrick Sutton, Senan Molony, Sandra Hurley, Helen Donohoe and Catherine Mac Eneaney.

I would also like to thank all my colleagues in RTÉ, in particular, Jon Williams, head of News and Current Affairs. For help in various ways with the book I would like to thank Bride Rosney, Gráinne Mooney, Oireachtas Library Services, Constance Cassidy and Professor David Farrell. I am very grateful to Su Watson who helped with the volume of interview transcripts, Natasha Fennell for her invaluable advice and Conor Nagle, commissioning editor at Gill Books, who saw the potential in *Madam Politician* and gave me great support and advice. I also appreciate the help from all the team in Gill Books.

Special thanks to my family – my mother Theresa and also Maira, Thomas, Céire and baby Sive. This book is dedicated to my late brother, Peter, and my late father, Tom.

Martina Fitzgerald

September 2018

Contents

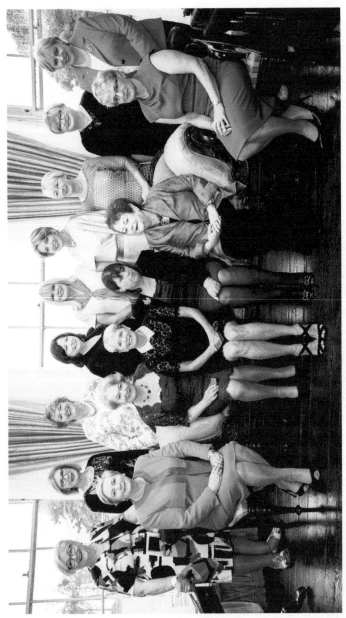

Lissadell House, Co. Sligo, July 2016: (*back row, left to right*) Niamh Bhreathnach, Jan O'Sullivan, Nora Owen, Mary Harney, Mary Mitchell O'Connor, Mary Coughlan, Mary Hanafin, Síle de Valera, Heather Humphreys; (*front row, left to right*) Frances Fitzgerald, Gemma Hussey, Constance Cassidy (owner of Lissadell House), Máire Geoghegan-Quinn, Mary O'Rourke, Katherine Zappone; (*note*) Joan Burton not in attendance; Regina Doherty and Josepha Madigan appointed senior ministers in 2017. (*Courtesy of James Connolly Photography*)

Introduction – Why So Few?

In July 2016, fourteen women from different backgrounds attended a dinner party in Co. Sligo. The women were members of one of Ireland's most exclusive clubs. What did they all have in common? The fourteen represent the majority of women who have served as senior ministers in Irish governments. The answer is not a punchline, it is a stark political reality.

A photograph of the dinner party taken in the summer of 2016 captures the jovial and celebratory mood of the evening. The fourteen women are sitting around a table, while three others (two are deceased and another was unable to attend) are missing from the photograph, one of many taken that night to capture the historic occasion. Their absence, however, could not mitigate the striking symbolism as dinner was served – all the Irish women who have been senior ministers since the first woman was appointed to government in 1919 could be seated around a single dining room table.

Since that evening in July 2016, two more women have been promoted to senior ministerial rank. But the numbers remain meagre, signifying missing female ministers and decades of missed opportunities. When Countess Constance Markievicz was appointed Minister for Labour in 1919, Ireland – then on the verge of achieving independence – could have been at the forefront in advancing women's representation in political life. In the initial two decades of the twentieth century, a woman's right to vote was taken seriously in many countries. In the United Kingdom, after a long and often fraught campaign, legislation was introduced in 1918 starting the process of women's suffrage. Irish women benefitted from these changes and in elections in the same year to the House of Commons, Markievicz became the first woman elected as a member of parliament (MP) at Westminster. At the time of her election, Markievicz was in prison in England. Having stood on an abstentionist platform, she and her Sinn Féin colleagues never took their seats in the House of Commons. Instead, the first Dáil was formed in Dublin. In April 1919, Markievicz was appointed a government minister, becoming the first Irish woman to hold a cabinet position.

Remarkably, it was sixty years before another woman was appointed to senior ministerial office in Ireland. In 1979, Máire Geoghegan-Quinn of Fianna Fáil was appointed Minister for the Gaeltacht, becoming the sole woman among her fourteen ministerial colleagues. This was an experience shared by several subsequent female ministers – Eileen Desmond (Labour, 1981–82), Gemma Hussey (Fine Gael, 1982–87), Mary O'Rourke (Fianna Fáil, 1987–92) and Geoghegan-Quinn herself again (1992–93). The official photographs of these governments – most of which are in black and white – not only record the historical occasions but freeze-frame periods in Irish society where men totally dominated positions of power.

It was not until the Fianna Fáil–Labour coalition was formed in January 1993 that two women sat around the cabinet table at the same time (Geoghegan-Quinn and Niamh Bhreathnach). More than twenty years after that underwhelming achievement, the figure doubled to four female ministers in 2014 – the highest level of female cabinet participation since the foundation of the state. The same number of female ministers was included in the governments formed by Enda Kenny in 2016 and Leo Varadkar in 2017. To put these numbers into perspective, of the 200 people appointed as senior ministers in Irish governments from 1919 up to September 2018, only nineteen have been women. In stark terms, around 90 per cent of all Irish senior ministers have been men; almost ten per cent have been women.[2] It has been a very long and painstakingly slow journey from 1919.

When it comes to the head of state role, the figures are somewhat better. Two of the nine presidents of Ireland since 1937 have been women – Mary Robinson and Mary McAleese. Robinson's election in 1990 made Ireland only the second country in Europe, after Iceland, to have a female head of state elected by popular vote. When McAleese became president in 1997, she became the first woman in the world to follow another woman into the office of elected head of state.[3] Yet, despite these achievements, it still took more than a half a century (1938–1990) for a woman to occupy the Irish presidency.

In the context of the 100th anniversary of Markievicz's appointment to cabinet in 1919, I wanted to write this book to tell the extraordinary stories of the seventeen surviving Irish women who were senior government ministers and the two women elected as president of Ireland (up to September 2018). These women do not form a homogenous group. There are commonalities and contradictions in their experiences that reflect their different backgrounds and views – as is the case in wider society. Their stories will resonate with those who love politics and also those who have little interest in politics, because their experiences encapsulate the social changes and challenges faced by many Irish women over the last few decades. Working as a female political correspondent in Leinster House, the 100th anniversary of Markievicz's appointment inspired me to tell the stories of the women who beat the odds and climbed to the top of the political system.

All nineteen women gave interviews specifically for this book so their voices are heard 'in the same room' for the first time. These stories reveal insights into their time on the campaign trail and on the corridors of power. Some stories are uplifting and inspiring, some amusing and collegiate; others are, quite frankly, depressing and bleak. Many of these female politicians pragmatically put some of their experiences down to the 'cut and thrust' of politics, which can be difficult for both men and women. But most of these women, who have served at the highest level in Irish political life, acknowledge they faced additional challenges – challenges that they believe discourage other women from participating in national politics.

❊ ❊ ❊

There was real historic symbolism in the fourteen female ministers gathering at Lissadell House in the summer of 2016. The property was the childhood home of Constance Gore-Booth (later Countess Markievicz). The dinner marked the 89th anniversary of her death. In media coverage of the event, Máire Geoghegan-Quinn recounted how, 'Constance Markievicz was a constant in my life because I was always being introduced when I was a minister as the first woman minister in the cabinet and of course I had to point out that this wasn't true.'[4]

When the invitation to the dinner arrived, it was not just the gap from Markievicz in 1919 to Geogheghan-Quinn in 1979 that forcefully struck former Tánaiste Mary Harney of the Progressive Democrats. When Bertie Ahern formed his first Fianna Fáil–

Progressive Democrats coalition in 1997, Harney was appointed to cabinet as Minister for Enterprise, Trade and Employment; she later served as Minister for Health and Children. By the time she left government in 2011, she held the distinction of being the longest-serving Irish female minister at cabinet. She was also the first woman to be appointed Tánaiste. Looking at the Lissadell dinner invitation, Harney counted out the number of women who might attend: 'I had never counted them before. I thought, my God, we haven't even hit twenty. It's incredible.'

All but one of the surviving senior women ministers eventually gathered at Lissadell House. One of the newest ministers, Mary Mitchell O'Connor of Fine Gael, who was Minister for Jobs, Enterprise and Innovation between 2016 and 2017, was instantly struck by the symbolism of the numbers as they sat down for dinner. 'That was a snapshot for me,' she says. The surviving women who are members of this exclusive ministerial club of nineteen describe the low number as 'shocking' (Gemma Hussey), 'pathetic' (Regina Doherty), 'outrageous' (Heather Humphreys), 'terrible' (Katherine Zappone), 'an incredible failure' (Joan Burton), 'disappointing' (Jan O'Sullivan) and 'beyond belief' (Frances Fitzgerald).

When they first entered Leinster House, many of these women had high hopes that their election was part of a process of finally advancing the position of women in parliament and in cabinet. Mary Coughlan was a senior minister in Fianna Fáil-led governments from 2002 to 2011. She was first elected to the Dáil in 1987 and says that if she had been asked at that time, she would have predicted that by the second decade of the 21st century, the representation of women in political life would be transformed: 'I would have been fully of the view that 50 per cent should have been in the House and 50 per cent should have been in the cabinet. And yet we didn't make it.' Her Fianna Fáil colleague Síle de Valera, who was Minister for Arts, Heritage, Gaeltacht and the Islands from 1997 to 2002, is in agreement: 'We have an awful long way to go. And I had hoped at this stage we would be much further on.' As emerges through the pages of this book, they were very much mistaken.

Most people are not conscious of the reality of the low numbers, according to Frances Fitzgerald, a senior Fine Gael minister from 2011 to 2017: 'They think because there's a couple of high-profile women, because you had President McAleese and President Robinson, that politics is nearly gender-neutral.' The reality, she points out, is so different. Fitzgerald, who also served as Tánaiste, is keen to correct the record about the level of women representation in Irish political life: 'It is majority male. There's more men called John or Michael than there are women. It's completely unfinished business. It's a completely unfinished democracy.' The Fine Gael politician sees serious implications for decision-making and policy formation: 'Women just aren't there. And if women aren't there, the men are making the decisions. That has the most profound implications on decisions, on priorities, on values.'

The politicians interviewed for this book share Fitzgerald's view that women's political representation has finally started to move in the right direction. Yet there is considerable impatience at the slow rate of progress. 'It's a long trek to have only that number,' Mary O'Rourke concedes. 'It should be more.' It certainly could have been more. O'Rourke sat at cabinet in Fianna Fáil governments led by Charles Haughey and Bertie Ahern (Taoiseach Albert Reynolds demoted her to a junior ministerial position). Looking back, she recalls 'loads of good women' in all the main parties who were never given the opportunity to serve.

Women have often been passed over for ministerial promotion in favour of male colleagues with less ability, according to Jan

O'Sullivan of Labour, Minister for Education and Skills from 2014 to 2016: 'There are some very able men who get to cabinet, and they should be in cabinet. But from time to time there are men who get to cabinet, when in my opinion there are women who aren't in cabinet who would be better.'

'You have to be an extraordinary female to get elected. You then had to be extraordinary to be appointed to cabinet,' says Mary Hanafin who served as a senior Fianna Fáil minister from 2004 to 2011. The former Labour leader Joan Burton holds the same view. As far as Burton is concerned, female politicians 'have to punch way above the level of their male colleagues'. Burton was a cabinet minister from 2011 to 2016 and served as Tánaiste for her last two years in government. She still sees a society in which 'any guy could be a minister or a Taoiseach', but a woman to be at cabinet – not to mind to Tánaiste or Taoiseach – is still considered 'a special event'.

The low numbers must be considered in a broader context, according to Gemma Hussey, a senior Fine Gael minister from 1982 to 1987. 'It's a chronicle of the development of a deeply conservative country, and that's the legacy,' Hussey believes. Political scientists Yvonne Galligan and Fiona Buckley argue that the dearth of women in positions of political power is only part of a wider pattern that showed the absence or under-representation of women in decision-making positions in Ireland generally.[5] After all, in the early 1970s, women had to accept lower rates of pay for doing the same work as their male colleagues and to give up their jobs in the public service after they got married. Broadcaster Marian Finucane once described such restrictions as 'Neanderthal now'.[6]

However, the conservatism that was so rooted in Irish society in the past cannot solely explain the lack of progress in the political sphere in recent times. As Irish society has modernised over the last thirty years, with a transformation in the role of women across all areas of life, the number of women in Dáil Éireann and, in particular, at the cabinet table has edged forward only gradually. The political digits have remained relatively stagnant, despite major changes in wider Irish society. In many respects Leinster House has almost resembled a parallel world. It is little wonder that Josepha Madigan of Fine Gael, the newest member of the ministerial club, talks about 'the stars aligning' in getting to the cabinet table. Madigan was appointed Minister for Culture, Heritage and the Gaeltacht in November 2017 and with her elevation the stars aligned for only the 19th woman in almost 100 years.

❧ ❧ ❧

At the cabinet table, female politicians view themselves as ministers and expect to be treated that way. But they operate in a world largely dominated by men. Until very recently, most senior civil servants in government departments were overwhelmingly male. Female ministers in the 1970s, 1980s and even in the 1990s headed departments run by male officials. As recently as 2007, only four women (25 per cent) occupied the top civil service position of secretary general, while a further twelve (13 per cent) held the position of deputy secretary general or assistant secretary. By January 2017, women held 29 per cent of secretary general positions and 28 per cent of deputy secretary general or assistant secretary positions.[7] In certain portfolios, female ministers walk into rooms that are still predominantly male.

The first woman to be Minister for Justice, Máire Geoghegan-Quinn, believes female ministers have to lay down the law from the outset to combat any unconscious bias. But she believes that it is equally important to be mindful of how this assertiveness is displayed. There are different views among those who have served at the highest level about publicly showing emotion – and this is not confined to Irish ministers or indeed to politics. In her memoir, former United States presidential candidate Hillary Clinton observes that successful women are often described as being angry, strident, feisty, difficult, irritable, bossy, brassy, emotional, abrasive, high maintenance or ambitious. These are predominantly negative terms. Clinton devotes a whole chapter to the general theme, such is its relevance for the experience of women in leadership roles.[8]

Many of the women who have served as senior ministers in Ireland believe showing emotion in public indicates vulnerability and can leave them open to the charge of being unprofessional or, worse still, hysterical. 'If you are emotional and sensitive and weepy, you are finished,' Mary Harney bluntly remarks. Others diverged from this view, with some believing it is more acceptable today and ultimately demonstrates heightened emotional intelligence. Others spoke about the expectation that female ministers should be more caring and softer in terms of the policy positions they adopt. Yet in the confines of the Dáil chamber, where all ministers spar with their opposition counterparts, most of these women believe there was little discrimination on account of their gender. They were subjected to the cut and thrust of politics – no different to their male colleagues and, certainly, no kinder.

That is not to say that blatantly sexist language has not been used in the Dáil chamber. 'That's women for you,' was how Taoiseach Albert Reynolds responded to Nora Owen of Fine Gael in 1992 when she heckled him during Leaders' Questions. This and other public comments have been called out for what they are. But other inappropriate remarks and unacceptable behaviour that female ministers have experienced have never been aired, let alone addressed, and many welcome the emergence of the international #metoo movement, which has prompted a greater awareness of the treatment of women in the workplace and, particularly, those in high-profile positions. Some of the comments and behaviour that Irish female politicians endured in the past would not be acceptable now. But, in truth, as their stories illustrate, they should not have been acceptable back then either.

Female ministers have also had to deal with public commentary, positive and negative, about their appearance. Many believe how they look is simply part of the job. They also acknowledge that the attention can sometimes be a political advantage amid a sea of 'men in grey suits'. There is, however, a general acceptance among the women interviewed of a double standard, with the appearance of female politicians sometimes dissected cruelly or subjected to hurtful commentary. While there have been some exceptions, they believe that the same treatment is generally not meted out to their male counterparts. This is again not confined to politics.

❀ ❀ ❀

To attain senior ministerial office requires getting the nod from the Taoiseach of the day or the leader of a party entering into a coalition government. Most politicians dream of a promotion; others expect it. Some have been known to demand elevation to cabinet and many have vented disappointment when overlooked. When Máire Geoghegan-Quinn was being appointed in 1979, she asked Fianna Fáil party leader Charles Haughey, 'Do you think I will be able?' Decades later, she still regrets that response. But Geoghegan-Quinn's question perhaps symbolises a lack of confidence that many women feel about their capabilities.

In determining the factors that influence cabinet appointments, Taoisigh tend to be cautious in their approach. In promotions to cabinet, they place a premium on loyalty, experience and length of service. They also tend to appoint people who are well known to them, which has meant that politicians who have served longer in the Dáil are generally appointed. Another part of the promotional equation is that dramatic changes during reshuffles and ministerial dismissals make political enemies of those demoted. [9] Given that the number of male TDs has historically been higher than those of female TDs, these factors combine to favour male politicians when it comes to deciding who gets a seat at cabinet.

Most of the women who have succeeded in attaining senior ministerial office agree there has been a level of stereotyping, with many women appointed to the so-called 'caring portfolios'. Forty-eight per cent of the women who have served in cabinet have been appointed to departments in the broadly defined social affairs area. When Mary Hanafin was appointed as Minister for Education in September 2004, she succeeded three other women who had held the same role (Gemma Hussey, Mary O'Rourke and Niamh Bhreathnach). Two of Hanafin's five successors in the job have been women. In all, of the nineteen women to have sat at cabinet, six have been Minister for Education, four have been Minister for Health while six have held the social affairs/social welfare portfolio at some stage.

On the other side of the ledger, seven women have served in economic briefs under the related departmental areas of business, enterprise, trade and innovation. Three of these female ministers, Fine Gael party colleagues Mary Mitchell O'Connor, Frances Fitzgerald and Heather Humphreys, have been appointed to the portfolio since 2016. The overall picture shows that 17 per cent of male ministers have held social affairs portfolios, while over half

(52 per cent) have served in economic and foreign policy briefs.[10] There are other notable trends when it comes to departmental allocations. Only one woman has occupied the senior ministerial role in the Department of Agriculture (Mary Coughlan) – that breakthrough came in 2004. As for the other political glass ceilings yet to be shattered, no woman has ever been appointed Minister for Finance or Minister for Defence or Minister for Foreign Affairs. These are the last male ministerial outposts.

'There's definitely a pigeonholing that takes place,' Hanafin says, 'and then suddenly there's great excitement when a woman goes into an economic ministry. And people say, "Oh look, wow." It's not in our ability, they kind of go, "Oh how did a woman get that sort of thing?" And that still happens, you know.' On her move from Education to Social Welfare in 2008, Hanafin says, 'Again it was one of those social kind of ones, where they will put a woman, you know.'

On the subject of female ministers being appointed to so-called 'caring' departments, Labour's Niamh Bhreathnach suspects 'it is probably because of our personalities, we actually do care a little bit wider or we have greater concerns'. The former Minister for Education references her previous and practical experience in the education sector as influencing her departmental allocation: 'I'm not saying it was a natural choice, but it wasn't like being landed with Foreign Affairs [so] that I would have to brief myself into.' She says the success of the previous female ministers in the department and their common career paths was also probably important: 'Gemma [Hussey] taught, but at a different level. But Mary O'Rourke taught and I taught. Career-wise we had had an experience. There were so few of us that it was easy to pigeonhole us – just to have a woman sitting at the cabinet table was an achievement.'

O'Rourke points out that the Departments of Education and Health are two of the biggest spending departments, although she concedes that they are also perceived as 'kind of womanly' departments. O'Rourke was Minister for both Education (1987–91) and Health (1991–92), and later Public Enterprise (1997–2002). From the outset of her political career in national politics in the early 1980s, she was very conscious of not being pigeonholed on gender grounds. As a result, she twice turned down the offer of having responsibility for women's affairs, once in opposition and later in government. Not long after first winning a seat in the general election in November 1982, which Fianna Fáil lost, Haughey rang the new Dáil TD. He was offering her a front-bench position as Fianna Fáil spokesperson on women's affairs and family law. She vividly remembers the conversation and her blunt response to her party leader: 'No, I don't want that, thank you.' Haughey wanted O'Rourke to shadow Nuala Fennell of Fine Gael, who had just been appointed a junior minister with the same responsibility.

'Imagine, I was a rookie TD, a month elected, here was the leader of my party ringing me. I often wonder where I got the nerve to say it,' she recalls. Haughey replied to O'Rourke, 'Oh, I see. And why not, pray?' The newly elected Longford–Westmeath TD answered, 'Because if you are a woman in women's affairs, I would be put in a cupboard with a label on the door, "Women's Affairs". So whenever contraception, divorce [are raised], pull Mary O'Rourke out to talk about those.' O'Rourke informed Haughey that she intended debating some of those social issues irrespective of any front-bench role.

Some female ministers reject the stereotyping of certain departments. Regina Doherty of Fine Gael says she wanted the Department of Social Protection position, which came her way in 2017. But others believe the appointments of Geoghegan-Quinn as the first woman to the Department of Justice (1993) and Coughlan as the first woman to the Department of Agriculture

(2004) show that female ministers can take on different portfolios outside the 'caring' departments. When Mary Harney was first appointed to cabinet, she headed the Department of Enterprise, Trade and Employment. She later became Minister for Health, which was her preference. 'There is pigeonholing,' she agrees. 'It's not just in politics, it's among the media as well.' Harney admits that, 'if the option was there to go to Finance, I would have loved it in different circumstances'. But, she recalls, as the leader of the smaller party in a coalition government with a significant gap in seat numbers with Fianna Fáil, the idea of Harney becoming Minister for Finance was not a runner.

But the Progressive Democrats leader still had considerable influence in the Department of Finance, given her long-standing friendship with Minister Charlie McCreevy – who got the position in 1997 – and their shared political and economic outlooks. She mentions the introduction of policies like the individualisation of the tax system as an example of her influence: 'I was very strong about that. A married woman went back to work and started paying tax at the marginal rate. It was crazy. So we [the Progressive Democrats] would have played a central role.'

On the odds of a woman attaining the top job in government, many of the female ministers believe, like Harney, it will happen but not for some time yet. Their collective view on this timeline may seem pessimistic, but many of these women believe this is anchored in political reality. Geoghegan-Quinn says her 'heart wants to see' a female Taoiseach in her lifetime. Humphreys agrees but admits, 'maybe not in my political lifetime'. O'Rourke is less confident about a woman occupying the Taoiseach's office in Government Buildings in the near future 'unless there's some big dramatic upheaval'. Nora Owen thinks a woman as Minister for Finance is more likely in the next decade than a woman as Taoiseach. Like many others, Hussey thinks the country is ready for a woman as Taoiseach but she says, 'whether the parties are ready for it now is another day's work'.

Despite the advancement of women's position in Irish society in recent decades, it is still harder for women to get what are considered 'the plum jobs', Frances Fitzgerald argues. The former Tánaiste believes there is no reason why a woman would not be Taoiseach or Minister for Finance, if the opportunity arose. But she points to the blockages in the political system: 'You first need to have more women in cabinet. And you need to build up the experience of being in cabinet. I certainly saw a difference in my performance in cabinet, from my first cabinet meeting to my last.'

Mary Hanafin holds the view that there might be a female Taoiseach before there is a female Minister for Finance. Her reasoning is based on the argument that the party membership has a role in the election of the former, while the Minister for Finance is appointed by the Taoiseach. 'It's not so much who selects it, I think it's just still seen as a job for a boy,' Hanafin says.

Joan Burton – who had expectations of the position in 2011 – hopes to see a woman serve as Minister for Finance, despite what she views as deeply entrenched views in the political system. 'It's probably oversold as being "too difficult" [for a woman] and because the thinking in parties is "Oh, only a man could do that". It's a go-to position because it's always been like this. "And women should mind the woman-style jobs."'

❧ ❧ ❧

Two of the nineteen women who served at cabinet have been leaders of their respective political parties (Mary Harney and Joan Burton), while six have served as deputy leaders (Mary O'Rourke, Mary Harney, Nora Owen, Mary Coughlan, Mary Hanafin and Joan Burton). Four women have served as Tánaiste

(Harney, Coughlan, Burton and Frances Fitzgerald), the second-highest ranking member of government. But there are significant gender gaps in leadership roles.

Harney was the first woman to be elected leader of a party in the Dáil when she became leader of the Progressive Democrats in 1993. She had been passed over for the role of deputy leader when the party was established in 1985, despite being a founding member and key driver behind the new venture. Instead, Des O'Malley – the Progressive Democrats leader – appointed Fine Gael TD Michael Keating as his deputy. Harney says getting the position 'would have been nice. But was I upset? No. I mean I saw the political necessity, you have to get somebody from Fine Gael.'

The Progressive Democrats leadership position fell vacant in 1993 but in a book published at the time, Harney ruled out running for the role.[11] 'Published just before I became leader then actually, ironically,' she remarks. Pressure from her party colleagues helped change her mind. 'I never saw myself in that position. First of all, I never thought Des would retire from the leadership as early as he did. I'm actually quite shy. And I'm very happy, you know, being the minister and being able to make decisions and make things happen. But then, I never saw myself in the overall leadership role. That was honest, that was the truth.'

Labour elected its first female leader when Joan Burton succeeded Eamon Gilmore in 2014. She also served as Tánaiste. Burton had previously been deputy leader of her party. Her party colleague Jan O'Sullivan says experience and ability were more important than gender in Burton securing these positions. But she recognises the symbolism involved: 'It's just a visual thing I think more than anything. I'm not sure that it in itself made a big difference, but it was important to women members in the party to be able to see that we had a female leader.' Burton says she was conscious that very few women had held such roles in Irish political life: 'You hope to be somebody who provides leadership in terms of how you do it yourself. But that you also open the road for other women to enjoy that position eventually, [that it] will become the norm.'

Burton had actually beaten O'Sullivan for the deputy leader position in 2007. O'Sullivan says her non-Dublin base and domestic considerations ultimately put paid to her leadership ambitions. 'I didn't feel I could be in Dublin for probably five days a week rather than the three days a week required of a TD or even of a deputy leader. Maybe that is a judgement that I made as a woman, maybe if I was a man I might have made a different judgement and said I will run for leader. But I had other responsibilities at the time.'

Women currently hold the leadership positions in two parties – Sinn Féin (Mary Lou McDonald) and the Social Democrats (Catherine Murphy, Róisín Shortall). None of these three women has, as yet, sat at cabinet. No Irish woman has ever led either of the two main parties, Fine Gael or Fianna Fáil. When Charles Haughey stood down as Fianna Fáil leader in January 1992, Mary O'Rourke contested the party leadership. She says Albert Reynolds already 'had all the votes wrapped up' as he swept to victory over her and the other candidate, Michael Woods. She frankly admits that there was 'no swell at all for me. Because I didn't have my heart in it. I never went out looking for votes.' There were, however, other more successful days for O'Rourke who was later appointed the first female deputy leader of Fianna Fáil by Bertie Ahern.

Interestingly, almost a quarter of a century since she secured that position, she feels the party was not ready at that point nor is it ready today for a female leader. 'I think in Fianna Fáil, it would be very, very hard for a woman to be leader. The voters of Fianna

Fáil around the country wouldn't be ready for it yet, I think.' This assessment is shared by another former senior Fianna Fáil politician, Máire Geoghegan-Quinn. Her verdict: 'I'm not sure the party still is ready.'

When Ahern won the Fianna Fáil leadership, succeeding Albert Reynolds in late 1994, Geoghegan-Quinn was his most likely opponent. The Galway West TD ultimately withdrew from the contest. She says neither the party nor herself was ready for her candidacy: 'I was so busy in the Department of Justice and I was totally concentrated on that, never thinking that the government was going to fall so quickly, never thinking that the party leader would be gone so quickly and that we would have this [leadership] competition.' Many close to Reynolds believed that had he survived a few more years as Taoiseach, Geoghegan-Quinn would have been well placed to succeed him. But with Reynolds's early resignation, this was not to be. Seán Duignan, who was government press secretary during the Fianna Fáil–Labour coalition, argued that she had 'singularly failed to build her own independent power base' within the party.[12] Geoghegan-Quinn accepts that Ahern had 'done his work and had the numbers'. She believes she also faced challenges as a female contender: 'It's one of the things that's very difficult for a woman. You can't be going into bars and buying drinks for fellas. You can't be in smoke-filled rooms and doing deals with fellas. And when I say fellas, I mean organisation members and all of that. But if you want to be the party leader you have to assiduously court people in a way. Meeting them and having coffee with them and discussing issues with them and doing deals with them. I'm not that kind of person.'

Mary Hanafin contested the Fianna Fáil leadership in 2011. She opted out in 2008 when Ahern stood down and Brian Cowen secured the position unopposed. 'It was the wrong time for me,' she says. Several supporters suggested she challenge but she accepted that Cowen 'was anointed at that stage so it wasn't going to happen'. When Cowen stood down amid political chaos in early 2011, Hanafin ran for the leadership against Micheál Martin, Brian Lenihan and Éamon Ó Cuív. Gender was not an issue: 'There was kind of a more rural–urban divide rather than a male–female divide so the issues weren't anything to do with being a woman or being a man,' she says. Like O'Rourke and Geoghegan-Quinn, Hanafin shares the view that it will be a very long time before a woman leads Fianna Fáil. 'Whoever she is, probably isn't there yet, you know, or maybe she's there, is new and hasn't made the mark yet,' Hanafin says. The former minister believes the Fianna Fáil organisation remains 'very male', that the party is 'not respectful enough of women' and has 'no supportive mechanism for women at all'.

Another member of the Fianna Fáil women's ministerial club, Síle de Valera also highlights the issue of political culture: 'There have been very few women there anyway. So we haven't reached a critical mass yet. And obviously to become leader of your party you need the votes. So it would be helpful if you had other support from women.' It does not, however, necessarily follow that women would vote en bloc for a female candidate. De Valera's grandfather, Éamon, was the first Fianna Fáil leader. She does not think 'Buying a pint would necessarily mean that you would make a good Taoiseach. But there is that culture there. It still remains. And what we need are more women to prove that they are more than equal to the task.'

No woman has ever even contested the leadership of the party in the history of Fine Gael. Gemma Hussey thought about seeking the position when Garret FitzGerald stood down in 1987. But she admits her unpopularity – associated with her tenure at cabinet when public expenditure reductions were the order of the day – lessened her appeal. She also believes gender was an issue:

'I didn't think the party was ready for a woman. I didn't think they would countenance a woman.'

Frances Fitzgerald has probably been best placed of any woman to run for the Fine Gael leadership. Yet following the resignation of Enda Kenny in 2017, she took a pragmatic decision when faced with the numerical reality of the nascent contest. In 1993 – not long after she was first elected to the Dáil – Fitzgerald expressed an interest in leading her party and being Taoiseach.[13] Reflecting on this early ambition, Fitzgerald says, 'in the meantime I got sort of more realistic. That was probably rather lightly said without much information or experience about it all. It didn't stay with me as a motivating force.' The decision not to run in the 2017 leadership contest was down to the reality of not having enough support to mount a serious challenge. She says she supported Leo Varadkar after careful consideration.

Fitzgerald's fellow Fine Gael TD Regina Doherty has ruled out running for the leadership of the party in the future due to family considerations. 'It would mean that I would genuinely have to turn my back on my parents, my husband and my four children. I'm too selfish to do that,' she says. Doherty believes these types of considerations are more likely to affect women than men in political life: 'I look at Leo and he works six-and-a-half days a week. I looked at Enda Kenny beforehand, and he worked seven days a week. He would phone his children every evening. I mean, I wouldn't be prepared to do that.' She admits that, 'there's a selfishness there that I happen to love my family more than I love my country. Not to be smart or anything about it, I wouldn't be prepared to give up that just to be the leader of a party or the leader of my country.'

Undoubtedly family life suffers when balancing a career in politics. All the women interviewed for this book accept there is a family–career trade-off. Burton acknowledges the sacrifices that families make in such circumstances: 'Most of the country's politicians, men and women, would not be where they are unless they had very understanding and supportive families and friends. And you miss being able to spend more time with your family.'

❧ ❧ ❧

The number of women who have served in cabinet since the foundation of the state reflects their under-representation in the Dáil. Any conversation about women in Irish politics cannot ignore this reality. The figures speak for themselves. From 1918 to 2018, 114 female TDs (9 per cent) have served in Dáil Éireann compared to 1,179 male TDs (91 per cent).[14] But if there are too few women in Dáil Éireann, it is not down to the voters. Research has shown that there is almost no evidence that women, as women, fare worse than men, or that voters discriminate for or against candidates on grounds of gender.[15] Many of the women appointed to cabinet point the finger of blame for the under-representation at the political parties. In the past women have not been nominated by the larger, more successful, parties. It is the smaller – and less successful – parties that are more likely to have women as candidates, partly for ideological reasons, but also because they have fewer incumbents and more rapid turnover.[16]

There has been a political awakening in terms of the need for more female TDs in recent years. The introduction of a 30 per cent gender quota for party candidates in the 2016 general election (increasing eventually to 40 per cent from 2023) is the direct result of the failure of political parties to voluntarily and actively promote women to run for office. Based on the evidence from other countries, Gemma Hussey has long been 'all in favour' of quotas. She believes the objective has to be more women in national politics: 'You do not want the parliament speaking and passing laws that don't reflect the population as a whole. It's a very faulty democracy where it isn't.' Few of the female ministers disagree.

There was little political resistance when the legislation providing for gender quotas was enacted in July 2012. It had the support of all political parties.[17] The statutory threat of a financial penalty was central to the legislative proposal. Parties that breach the quotas stand to lose half the public funding available to them for the full duration of the parliamentary term following the election. On the basis of the 2016 general election, it has proven to be a very effective stick to force the parties to act. 'Unless you direct parties to do what we directed them to do under the gender legislation, I think we probably could have carried on the way we have always carried on,' Regina Doherty says.

The general election in 2016 was a watershed in terms of the level of female representation in the national parliament: 35 women were elected to the Dáil. This was an increase of 40 per cent on the number of women elected in 2011 and although it is still far from gender parity, this means that 22 per cent of TDs in the current Dáil are women, the highest proportion of female TDs in the history of the state.[18] This historically high level of female members of parliament is unimpressive when compared with some other European countries at the start of 2018 – Sweden (44 per cent), Finland (42 per cent), Spain (39 per cent), Belgium (38 per cent) and the United Kingdom (32 per cent). In fact, Ireland was ranked 78th out of 193 countries in terms of female representation in January 2018.[19] So while the introduction of gender quotas along with stiff financial penalties in 2016 has rightly been lauded, it should really be seen as a starting point.

Interestingly, some of the women who have served in cabinet were strong opponents of gender quotas in the past. Others spent years actively advocating and campaigning for their introduction.

Their contrasting positions reflect the broad spread of views on the use of quotas. When the gender-quota legislation debate took place, Niamh Bhreathnach was able to point to how they had been instrumental in the early stages of her political career. The introduction of two reserved places for women in the 1980s ensured she got onto Labour's national executive. 'They are very crude,' she concedes, adding, 'but nobody has come up with anything that will make the same difference.' Nora Owen says her 'verdict on quotas is still out' but she is not in favour of getting rid of them as she believes they rightly forced the political parties to act. Owen wants to see more analysis on their effectiveness as she believes many of the women who won seats in 2016 were already on the road to election while others fall into the Independent category and were therefore outside gender quotas.

The two former female presidents, along with the majority of the women who have held senior ministries, are hugely supportive of the introduction of quotas for general elections. Heather Humphreys gives this assessment: 'I always believed that you get a job because you are the best person for the job, regardless of whether you are a man or a woman. But I do think that the quotas served a very useful purpose. Because it got more women on the ticket and now we have more women than ever before elected to this Dáil.' Indeed, Katherine Zappone, an Independent TD who was appointed as Minister for Children and Youth Affairs in 2016, would now like quotas to rise to 50 per cent of female candidates being nominated.

Other women, previously uncomfortable with the idea, have since been persuaded by the merits of a gender-quota system, including a number of former Fianna Fáil ministers. Máire Geoghegan-Quinn says she was always against quotas but now accepts that they 'delivered in the last election and they have put a focus in every single political party now. I see it in Fianna Fáil,

I see it in my own constituency, people are saying, "Oh God, we have to have a woman on the ticket." And now they are actually looking, not just for a woman, they are looking now for a woman who can make a difference and who can deliver votes.' If her party colleague Síle de Valera had been asked ten years ago about gender quotas, she admits she would not have been in favour of them. But she now accepts that quotas may be the only approach to increasing women's representation: 'I think maybe to give things a kick-start, maybe quotas are necessary. I was hopeful things would change. But they have changed so slowly, maybe we do need that kick-start.'

Mary Hanafin agrees: 'I was always 100 per cent against them. But I have to say, I thought it was clever linking it to the financial contributions of the parties. It forced the parties to find people.' However, while Hanafin favours the current system 'for a couple of elections, I wouldn't do it forever'. She would stop at the 40 per cent quota: 'I would use it for a few elections to try and get people in and get them established. But they are not going to do it simply by turning around the week before the nominations close and grabbing a few women and nominating them.' Mary Coughlan believes the 'financial penalty has made people buck up'. From a position of been 'very anti-quotas because then you were just picked because you were a woman', Coughlan now accepts that 'it's a good idea that you have to have so many women putting their name forward'.

Mary O'Rourke is a lone voice among the women interviewed in her absolute opposition to gender quotas: 'I always believe women should be supported and put forward and I would be out for more women in politics, but not the gender quota. That is so wrong.' O'Rourke is adamant she is not for turning: 'I will never change it on quotas because it's not fair. It's not fair to a man or a woman. You should go on your merit.'

Nevertheless, gender quotas are here to stay and will be part of the political architecture in Ireland for the foreseeable future. Given the importance of local involvement as a foothold to national politics, it is hardly surprising that the debate has extended to seeking the introduction of gender quotas at local-government level. Eighty-three per cent of the women elected in the 2016 general election were councillors at some stage in their political careers.[20] A positive report card on gender quotas in national politics has most likely helped the case for introducing them in local elections but their introduction is by no means guaranteed.

There is also the question of gender quotas for cabinet positions. Reflecting on the developments since 1919, when Ireland led the way internationally in appointing a female minister, the legacy of successive Irish governments has been exceptionally disappointing. Women's groups and some politicians argue the parties cannot be left to their own devices and that another interventionist approach may be necessary.[21] Yet, surprisingly, the appetite for gender quotas at cabinet level seems to be lacking among most of the women who have attained senior office.

Nora Owen opposes the idea of a quota system at cabinet, believing that it 'would mean that some very good men would be passed over, and that's not fair either'. Niamh Bhreathnach, a long-time supporter of quotas in politics, is opposed to them being imposed on cabinet nominations: 'You are a minister then. You are not a woman, you are not a man.' Máire Geoghegan-Quinn is equally unconvinced as, she says, at cabinet a Taoiseach needs to consider the best 'skillsets' to run the country. She is also wary of the idea of politicians being appointed to departments where they have a professional advantage, such as a teacher in education, a doctor in health and an architect in housing: 'I feel, as a teacher myself, you bring a certain unconscious bias to the area of education that you know best. So if you have let's say a primary school teacher as Minister for Education, which we have had, I think, in the past, their natural focus in the department is going to be on, you know, putting money into making improvements in primary education.'

The two former presidents also have the same view on this issue and interestingly, it is the minority one among the female senior office holders. Mary Robinson points to Canada, where half the cabinet are women. 'There's a whole prioritising of that being normal and now let's see how we have to adjust our system,' she says, adding: 'I think it's a real breakthrough when a prime minister says half my cabinet will be women.' Mary McAleese also favours gender quotas in cabinet: 'Absolutely, we need more women.'

Of those female politicians in favour of gender quotas for cabinet, some believe such an approach could only be considered for ministerial office when women occupy half of the Dáil seats. The introduction of 40 per cent gender quotas for candidates in general elections from 2023 onwards is widely seen as another significant turning point in changing the gender landscape of the Dáil, thereby placing greater pressure on future Taoisigh to have full gender balance in ministerial appointments.

Gemma Hussey is one of those who believes the quota in cabinet should be the same as the quota in the Dáil: 'I don't see why a leader should be worried about having a quota for cabinet, which would be the same as the quota for the Dáil. It only follows logically.' Joan Burton shares that view: 'I want to hear every party saying, if we are in government it's going to be a government of 50:50, with a minimum of 40 per cent women, 40 per cent men. And after that it's strictly 50:50. But I want to hear all the party leaders say, it's my objective, should I be in a position to be a member of the cabinet, to have 50 per cent of my team be women.'

But two women who, like Burton, served as Tánaiste, disagree. Frances Fitzgerald believes the answer lies in ensuring more women are elected to the Dáil, thereby providing a greater choice for cabinet promotions: 'Sometimes Taoisigh get criticised unfairly because they don't have the numbers of women. I think you have to take positive action, all things being equal you have to appoint a woman if you want to get the balance. [But] not at cabinet, no. Because you have to get that mix at cabinet, and you do have to be aware of experience and expertise, and the balance of what you are trying to achieve in your cabinet.' Mary Harney agrees: 'I don't think it's practical, to be quite frank with you. I actually take the view that the best people should be put in the best jobs, regardless of women or men. And the best should apply to men – sometimes it's only applied to women.'

❋ ❋ ❋

Over time the political profile and ideology of the women who serve in cabinet may evolve. In the future, we may see female politicians from Sinn Féin, the Green Party, Social Democrats or Solidarity–People Before Profit attain senior ministerial office. Whatever their political hue, more public and media attention is certain to be focused on the actual number of women appointed to cabinet after future electoral cycles. It is now part of the political conversation and commitments will be sought although they cannot always be guaranteed from political leaders. A study of ministerial appointments to governments across seven countries found that a personal pledge by those in charge may be one of the biggest forces in improving gender equality. Researchers suggest that such a pledge is powerful because those who make it are in a position to ensure change happens, and will also be held accountable if they fail to act.[22] However, this has not been the experience of female politicians in Ireland – in late 2014, Taoiseach Enda Kenny promised that half of the positions in cabinet after the subsequent general election would be filled by women, but appointed just four after the 2016 general election. The Fine Gael leader may have been hampered by the make-up of the minority coalition and the routine political considerations of geography and seniority. Ultimately, however, the number of women at cabinet did not increase as promised.

Future appointments will come under intense scrutiny. Just as groups such as the Women's Political Association (WPA) advocated for greater female representation in the 1970s and 1980s, other organisations with similar intent have now emerged inside and outside of Leinster House. For example, Women for Election is advocating for change and on a practical level has provided courses for female candidates. Inside the confines of Leinster House, female politicians formed a women's caucus in 2017. Gender quotas coupled with public and media scrutiny and the campaigns of advocacy groups are all aligning at a time in which an awareness of the importance of involving women in politics is gaining traction internationally. Timing, as everyone knows, is important in politics.

The question remains – by 2025 or 2030, how many dinner tables will be needed at a social event to accommodate the women who have served at cabinet in Ireland, and how many women will be sitting around these tables? Trick questions and tricky ones for political leaders. Irrespective of who is in power, the answer lies in whether the political will exists to change the seating arrangements.

1

ELECTIONS – CLIMBING THE POLITICAL LADDER

They were pretty clear that the place of the woman was in the home.

MARY ROBINSON

Mary Robinson remembers getting 'quite a lot of pushback' when she was seeking to win a Dáil seat in the 1970s and 1980s. Politics aside, she got a lot of flak for being a mother who was seeking election. 'You should be at home minding the child, not coming around,' she remembers some voters bluntly remarking.

The political and social climate of the time is important in understanding the challenges she and other women faced on the campaign trail. In the early 1970s, Irish women had to give up their jobs in the public service when they got married. They had to accept lower pay for doing the same work as men. They could not buy contraceptives. They could not refuse to have sex with their husbands. The list of what today seem incredibly anti-women policies and attitudes went on and on. The position of Irish women was aptly captured in a 'job description' printed on the cover of the magazine *Bread and Roses*, produced by women in UCD in the mid-1970s. It depicted a cartoon of a woman calling out 'Girls! Looking for a career? Become a housewife!!!'[23]

Against this backdrop, female politicians were, as Nora Owen, a former Fine Gael Minister for Justice, puts it, 'a rare species'. In 1973, there were just four female TDs in the Oireachtas. To use Frances Fitzgerald's political barometer, the seven TDs named Michael in the Dáil at the time outnumbered the female representation in the chamber. Four years later, in 1977, the number of female TDs elected had risen to six – but the number of TDs named Michael was double this. Inside and outside Leinster House, there were restrictions on the role and influence of women in Irish society. The women who pounded the pavements seeking election in the 1970s and 1980s were trailblazers. Their experiences reveal much about the challenges and changes women faced in Irish society and why so few women were appointed to cabinet during this period.

❧ ❧ ❧

Mary Robinson's greatest triumph at the ballot box was in the presidential election in 1990. Prior to her historic election as Ireland's seventh head of state, she had mixed fortunes at the ballot box. She was first elected to Seanad Éireann in 1969 in the restricted constituency of Dublin University. She held the seat at six subsequent elections, her political career in the upper chamber spanning twenty years. She had, however, less success in seeking a Dáil seat, enduring defeat in the 1977 and 1981 general elections as a Labour candidate.

When Robinson ran for a Dáil seat in Dublin West in 1981, she was pregnant with her third child. It was a big decision to contest the election: 'I had been very much encouraged by the Labour Party – I mean, really pursued – to stand for election. I was at an early stage of pregnancy. I didn't know when the election would be called, but it was likely to be in May when my baby was due. And of course, this is what happened. Aubrey was born on 3 May, and the election was called on 20 May.' Polling day was set for 11 June 1981.

Robinson went on the campaign trail with a newborn baby and had to make practical arrangements for breastfeeding. The main thing 'was to find safe houses' to feed her son. She recalls the journalist Nell McCafferty spending a day with her out canvassing: 'She was fascinated because she was talking to me while I was feeding. And when I finished on one side and I was about to shift to the other side, she says, "Do you feel empty, Mary, do you feel empty on that side?" And I thought, oh my God, she's going to write about this.' Practical issues aside, Robinson also faced social judgements on her decision to contest the election. Knocking on doors in Ballyfermot and other areas in the five-seat Dublin West constituency, Robinson was confronted by voters who were 'pretty clear that the place of the woman was in the home.' Surprisingly such comments were made by men and women.

It had not been a great deal easier on her first attempt to be elected in 1977, when she faced a campaign to blacken her name. On the eve of polling day, a notice was pushed through letterboxes in Dublin–Rathmines West, where she was a Labour candidate. It claimed she was benefiting financially from contraceptive prescriptions issued by a well-known pharmacy firm that bore her surname but to which she had no association. Robinson had gained national notice as a reforming liberal politician and lawyer on equality and social issues, including the availability of contraceptives. As contraceptives were banned in Ireland at the time, the contents of the leaflet were highly controversial. She still believes the smear campaign – by unknown political opponents – 'did some damage' to her performance on election day. She never found out who was responsible but believes they were distributed 'at a pivotal moment' of the campaign. Ultimately, she views the outcome as a blessing in disguise: 'I don't think I would have done a very good job. And [being elected to the Dáil] probably would have turned me off politics altogether.' Robinson was not in favour of wheeling and dealing: 'I was never of the "I will fix it for you" because I didn't agree with "I will fix it for you" sort of politics.'

Thirteen years later as a presidential candidate, Robinson faced further smears. During the campaign in 1990, she remembers one Roman Catholic priest labelling her a 'Marxist, lesbian bitch'. Rumours about the state of her marriage, which had first circulated when she was trying to win a Dáil seat, also resurfaced: 'There were a lot of rumours […] that Nick and I were divorcing.' She found the gossip about 'a sham marriage' during the presidential campaign very hurtful. Robinson believes such rumours were deliberately spread but she never found out where they originated.

In all her electoral contests – Seanad, Dáil and presidential – Robinson was backed by female supporters on the campaign trail. In her first Seanad contest in 1969, most of the women carried out an unglamorous but essential task – they 'licked and sticked' stamps on envelopes stuffed with election literature to be sent to voters.

Robinson was a reluctant presidential candidate in 1990. The idea first arose when the attorney general at the time, John Rogers, asked to see her. Rogers was a confidant of Labour leader Dick Spring and a legal colleague of Robinson's at the bar. Initially, she thought Rogers wanted to discuss a personal issue: 'I thought he had a family problem to be honest, when he asked to see me in my home, and that he was going to ask me as a friend to take his case.' Rogers, however, had an entirely different proposition: 'I hadn't ever thought about being president. I was very surprised and not very enthusiastic. And he could tell from my face that I looked as though I was going to say "no".'

Encouraged by her husband, Nick, Robinson quickly came around to the idea of being a presidential candidate. But she had no expectation of becoming the next occupant of Áras an Uachtaráin: 'I was very aware that I had no real prospect of winning. I mean, the bookmakers made me 100/1 against.' While Labour provided the route to her nomination as a presidential candidate, Robinson was adamant from the outset that she would contest as an Independent. Despite being promoted by Spring, her candidacy faced opposition within Labour, including from Michael D. Higgins, who later also became head of state. Higgins favoured Noël Browne, who had been a Clann na Poblachta minister in the first inter-party government in 1948 and subsequently joined a number of parties, including the Labour Party. There was some tension during a campaign visit to Higgins's base in Galway: 'He didn't warm to me. I'm not trying to make an issue of it now, because, I mean, we are friends for a long time [but] he was one of those who regretted that I had got the nomination and not Noël Browne.'

Having secured the nomination, Robinson was out early on the campaign trail. While she was well known in political and legal circles, she was far from a household name: 'I could walk down the street and people didn't know who I was. I was not known.' Previously in her career she looked to her father for inspiration and 'had tended to slightly model myself on my father, who was a shy, professional doctor [...] very good at his job, but slightly shy. Very good with people, at a certain level.' As a presidential candidate, she looked to her mother as a role model: 'My mother was a terribly warm, open person. And what I found was that in standing for the presidency, you actually had to open yourself. And once I did it, I realised this is great. This is the way I want to be.'

Several years after the end of her term as president, Robinson was in the United States giving a talk in Idaho when a young Irish woman approached her: 'When I finished the talk, I saw this youngish woman walking, striding up. I actually came down from the platform, because she had her hand out. She clearly wanted to shake my hand. [The woman said] "I want to shake your hand, you were my first vote. I was nineteen years old at the time, and when I told my father, he nearly killed me."'

❧ ❧ ❧

Nora Owen also had to juggle being a mother and a Dáil candidate in the early 1980s and it was often a matter of comment on the hustings. From a practical perspective, she was prepared for the challenge of running for election, having had three children under the age of seven when she was elected a Fine Gael councillor. Her successful run in the 1981 general election required her husband Brian becoming 'a full-time babysitter'. It was a team effort. He started work quite early and would arrive home mid-afternoon, which allowed her go knocking on doors. Some voters in Owen's Dublin North constituency posed questions about her domestic arrangements: 'I would get people saying, "Who is minding the children?" Others would remark, "Aren't you a great girl to be standing, and you with small children? You know, it's going to be very busy."'

Fine Gael ran two candidates in Dublin North in 1981, the outgoing TD John Boland and Owen. The other six candidates in the three-seat constituency were men. Owen's status as the only woman on the ballot paper was not unusual at that time. It was the norm.

In seeking a Fine Gael nomination in 1981, Owen had to seriously consider the impact on family life if she won a Dáil seat: 'I knew if I did by chance get elected, I was going to have to make big changes in my household, from the point of view of childminding.' The ad hoc arrangements she had put in place since winning a seat on Dublin County Council in 1979 were unlikely to be sufficient for a career as a national politician. The recruitment of a housekeeper was discussed. She wonders if such domestic considerations ever entered the minds of male candidates at the time: 'I don't know whether a young man, a father, has to think in any way about, "Well, I won't stand or I will stand" [because of childminding and housekeeping issues],' Owen says.

❖ ❖ ❖

Male candidates did not have to face the same barrage of negativity that women faced on the hustings as a result of their decision to stand for elected office. 'You should be at home and not be taking a job from a man,' one woman told Gemma Hussey, who was a first-time Dáil candidate for Fine Gael at the 1981 general election. Hussey, who served in cabinet from 1982 to 1987, still remembers her response: 'I just said to her, "Look, I will do my best. It's all I can do. I'm not taking a job from anybody."' As one of the founders of the Women's Political Association (WPA), Hussey was well able to bat away such remarks.

The WPA emerged in Ireland in the 1970s to encourage more Irish women to stand for election at a time when women's groups internationally were becoming increasingly vocal about equality issues. A membership form for the WPA in the early 1980s put it plainly: 'Our country is losing out on the use of one of its greatest natural resources – women.' The leaflet emphatically declared that 'nothing will change until women represent women in sufficient numbers at all levels of public life'. The WPA's stated target was a 'minimum of 40 per cent representation at all levels of policy-making'.[24] Four decades later, that goal has not been achieved.

Looking back, Hussey says she and her WPA colleagues 'got very fired up and we went around the place making speeches. The women's movement was kind of gathering pace. The whole thing was to say that you can't have a proper democracy without women being strongly represented. And in Ireland, at the time, we had hardly any women at all [in political life].' Hussey and other WPA members felt the need to 'talk up' their efforts: 'We used to tell the most terrible lies. I remember telling a lie to one journalist in RTÉ. [He asked] "How many members have you got?" "Oh, about 1,000," I said, bold as brass. We had about thirty. And they were mostly in Dublin. But we decided we would go for broke.'

The WPA travelled the country promoting the position of women in Irish political life. Hussey recalls one trip to Dundalk in the company of Nuala Fennell – later a Fine Gael TD – and the journalist Nell McCafferty from Co. Derry: 'I was driving, and it was November, and it was dark and cold. And Nell kept saying, as we got nearer the border, "For God's sake, Gemma, don't be getting lost now or I will be kneecapped. The Provos [the Provisional Irish Republican Army] don't like me."'

The meetings were as eventful as the trips. Hussey and Fennell were left somewhat terrified of McCafferty's forthright personality, which was on display that evening when she decided to confront an audience at a packed school hall in Dundalk that included local politicians and nuns: 'The three of us got up. Luckily, I spoke first. That was grand. Nuala then spoke and then Nell got up. Nell gave us the history of how the bra was invented, how it went through in its various stages, that you were either sticking out or flat or going sideways. And this was all to do with what society thought of women at the time. She went into very graphic descriptions of what the bras did. In the middle of her speech, some nuns in the front row got up and walked out. It was kind of a religious walk-out, because Nell had been so irreverent.'

It was soon time for Hussey to practise what she preached. Her entry into political life began when she ran for the Seanad on the National University of Ireland (NUI) panel in 1977 as an Independent candidate. She looked to her female friends for support: 'They were fantastic. They wrote letters by hand to every single graduate they had ever met.' Many of these women also backed her when she ran unsuccessfully as a Fine Gael candidate in Wicklow in the 1981 general election and again in February 1982 when she won a Dáil seat for the first time. These women canvassed wearing yellow stickers displaying the slogans of the WPA: 'Who is your Woman? Why not a Woman? Vote for the Woman.' As Hussey recalls, not everyone in Fine Gael was impressed: 'You see the WPA, which was still in existence at this stage, they would send down people to canvass for me as well but you weren't supposed to get somebody to canvass for you that wasn't a party member. And these women, none of them were party members. [But they were] doing it for women.'

Hussey's statement isn't just a soundbite. The WPA played a practical role in kickstarting the political career of another future Minister for Education around this time. Niamh Bhreathnach, who was first elected to the Dáil for Labour in 1992, started attending WPA meetings in the 1970s. She remembers meeting women like Nuala Fennell, Monica Barnes and Frances Fitzgerald (who at various times served as Fine Gael TDs) at these events: 'They were very politically sophisticated in comparison to me. I probably went for about a year, once a month, I think. And one night they said, "What are you all really sitting for? You should join political parties."' Each of the main political parties made recruitment presentations at WPA meetings. Bhreathnach was energised by

Labour's advocacy for reform in the areas of divorce and family planning, issues that she considered 'rights for women'.

She joined Labour in 1976: 'My mother went to her grave without understanding why I joined the Labour Party.' For Bhreathnach, 'it was about finding an outlet for my concern about creating an environment in which women's voices would be heard'. She quickly realised, however, that women in Labour in the 1970s and 1980s also had to fight to get their voices heard. 'When you went to [Labour] Conference, they were all men on the stage. The party's women's council didn't meet in head office because they didn't really let the women in.'

Women also had to campaign to get representation on the party's administrative council. As Bhreathnach recalls, 'We had to put that to Conference. And two of our own women spoke against it.' Despite this ironic turn of events, the women's council eventually secured two reserved places on the administrative council and Bhreathnach was elected to one of these positions. She has been a strong supporter of gender quotas since then. In the Spring Tide general election of 1992, when the number of Labour TDs jumped from fifteen to thirty-three under the leadership of Dick Spring, Bhreathnach won a seat in Dún Laoghaire. She holds the distinction of being one of only six TDs to be appointed to cabinet on first arriving in the Dáil, serving as Minister for Education until 1997.

❧ ❧ ❧

Women faced similar challenges and battles in other political parties in the 1970s and 1980s to ensure their voices were heard. The attitude of some senior party officials may explain in part why so few women got involved in politics, let alone sought public office.

Former Fianna Fáil Minister for Justice Máire Geoghegan-Quinn was encouraged that women got actively involved in her by-election campaign in 1975: 'There were about five or six women locally, who had never got involved before but were very Fianna Fáil. They went out of their way. They canvassed, did all sorts of stuff for me to get to know people.' But after the election, their work was not recognised within the party: 'When the election was over and I went to my first cumann [branch] meeting in that area, I walked in the door and I was surrounded by a sea of men.' As the newly elected TD, Geoghegan-Quinn addressed the meeting and thanked everyone for their support during the by-election campaign. She mentioned her hope for the continued involvement of her female supporters in the local party organisation: 'I said, "I hope that when I come to my next cumann meeting that I will see some, if not all, of the women who worked so hard for me and for the party during the election campaign."' The new TD was quickly put in her place – she remembers the unofficial rules of the cumann being firmly laid down: 'Now, now, girlie. It's enough – we have you, a woman as a TD, without having women at meetings. There's no place for women here.' The comments were made by 'the oldest man in the room, who was the president of the [local] organisation, which was an honorary position at the time [...] He was genuine. He wasn't annoyed. He was just stating something, which to him was a matter of fact.' Geoghegan-Quinn pressed the issue again: 'But what about all these women who did so much good work during the three weeks of the campaign?' The older man's reply was short and to the point: 'Ah, that's fine. They will do it for the next election too, but they're not going to be in at the cumann meetings.' Nobody else at the meeting challenged this or spoke up in defence of the women.

Today such comments would most likely trigger a number of responses – widespread condemnation, protests and the possibility of legal action or all of the above. There is an irony in that on one hand women were being obstructed in getting involved at the most basic level in local politics, while on the other hand the same party machine had actively campaigned for a female candidate to run for national politics. Party officials specifically sought out Geoghegan-Quinn to run for the Dáil in 1975. She is one of several women with family roots in the political system to have served in cabinet. Her father, Johnny Geoghegan, won a Dáil seat in Galway West in 1954. He was promoted from the backbenches to parliamentary secretary (junior minister) in 1970 during the political turmoil of the Arms Crisis, which saw two Fianna Fáil ministers dismissed for their alleged involvement in the illegal smuggling of arms to the Irish Republican Army (IRA) in Northern Ireland. He held the position until Fianna Fáil lost office three years later.

Following his death in January 1975, attention quickly moved to the impending by-election. In Fianna Fáil circles, there was interest in the idea of a Geoghegan family member being the party's candidate. At the time, Geoghegan-Quinn was newly married and the mother of a young baby. She had no interest in embarking on a political career. However, the decision was in effect made for her and she effectively became a bystander in the process: 'I'm in my mother's house – a Saturday or a Sunday afternoon – the doorbell rings. The chairman and the secretary and some other members of the hierarchy in the party in Galway arrive. They go in with my mother into the sitting room. I'm in the kitchen making tea for them. And the next thing, my mother comes out and she said, "We want you to come inside." They thought I would be the best person and the best known and blah, blah, blah ...' And so the political career of the second Irish woman appointed to cabinet and a future Minister for Justice began.

In seeking the party's nomination, Geoghegan-Quinn received a warm welcome from Fianna Fáil members in Galway West. But, she remembers, there were doubts about how a young mother could devote the necessary time to a political career: 'Everywhere I went, there was a great welcome but at the same time people were saying, "Your father was such a fantastic TD. He was available seven days a week and all the rest of it. How can you do that? You are a young married woman and you have a baby." So I had to do a convincing job on that.' While Geoghegan-Quinn was a bystander in the decision to contest the by-election, on the party hustings she actively framed a response to counter any doubts: 'I said, you know, I will probably never be as good as my father. I won't do things the way he did. I will do them differently, but hopefully I will do them just as well, and I will get the same results at the end of the day.'

Having secured the Fianna Fáil nomination, she faced similar questions from the electorate in Galway West about combining the roles of mother and politician. On the doorsteps canvassing for the March 1975 by-election, she advised voters: 'I will be available six days a week to do whatever needs to be done. But I will be taking Sunday off. That will be my day off. But apart from that, I said, you will get my utmost attention.' Geoghegan-Quinn points out that her male counterparts did not face similar scrutiny: 'You can be certain they didn't ask any of the men. In those days – and, indeed, very often nowadays too – you still have a situation where the woman has the job outside the home, but she's also the homemaker when she comes home in the evening. She still has to do the washing and the cleaning and the cooking, as well as having a job outside the home. And so, in that sense, not an awful lot has changed since my time.'

❧ ❧ ❧

Nearly half a century since Máire Geoghegan-Quinn's election, the number of women working outside the home and in the national parliament has increased. However, the number of women in the Dáil has come from a very low base. Just four of the 144 TDs that were elected in 1973 were women – 3 per cent of the total. When Geoghegan-Quinn retained her seat in the 1977 general election, she was joined on the Fianna Fáil backbenches by Síle de Valera, the 22-year-old granddaughter of the party's founder, Éamon de Valera. Geoghegan-Quinn was elevated to cabinet a little over two years later; de Valera's ministerial promotion came two decades later. At the outset of their careers in Irish national politics, these two women shared similar backgrounds and experiences: professionally, both had qualified as teachers; politically, both came from 'political dynasties'. They also worked – and progressed – in a male-dominated environment that was Irish politics in the late 1970s.

Like Geoghegan-Quinn, de Valera grew up in a political family. De Valera was as close as its gets to Fianna Fáil royalty. Her grandfather, Éamon, had been party leader from 1926 to 1959. He had served both as Taoiseach and as president. Politics was the family's profession. As de Valera recalls, 'We were always encouraged around the table just to sit and discuss issues. And it didn't matter if you were the only person with an opposite view around the table, as long as you could argue that succinctly. And that was a great training for debate and a great training for politics and for life generally.' While a student of history and politics at UCD, her father offered some advice: 'Síle, it's all very well looking at politics in a theoretical point of view. But why don't you join a political party and see what the practical side is like?'

De Valera's grandfather, who completed a second term as president in 1973, died in August 1975. But there was still a family link to political life. Vivion de Valera, an uncle, was still a TD when de Valera was contemplating getting involved in party politics. Surprisingly, given her family background, it was not an automatic choice to join Fianna Fáil: 'I know people would say, "Oh well, you would join Fianna Fáil, wouldn't you?" [But] it wasn't just Fianna Fáil I was looking at. I also looked at the Labour Party.' In the end, de Valera opted for Fianna Fáil based on what she describes as the party's 'very broad sense of what republicanism is, in the social and political sense'.

De Valera was nominated to contest Dublin County Mid in the 1977 general election and concedes that 'name recognition' was important in helping her win a seat. But she says this type of recognition can only take a candidate so far: 'You may be elected because your name is known on your first election, but after that you are on your own. You have to prove yourself capable of doing the job. It's not just a question of sentimentality that you are voted in. It certainly would be of tremendous help the first time. But after that I think it would be very unfair to suggest […] that you could coast on that for your political life.' This was certainly true for de Valera. She won a seat in the Fianna Fáil landslide election in 1977, then failed on her next three attempts before returning to the Dáil in 1987 for the Clare constituency where her grandfather had held a seat for some forty years. She retained her seat in the four subsequent general elections until her retirement from politics in 2007. So while name recognition was helpful, it also had its limitations.

Family name aside, de Valera shares much in common with other women who sought elected office during this period. As a woman running for the Dáil, she was among a distinct minority. But for her, the focus was not just on her gender – she felt there was also a particular concentration on her age. Arriving into Leinster House in 1977 at the age of 22, de Valera was the youngest TD in the new Dáil. This didn't go unnoticed: '[There was] more negativity towards the fact that I was young, more than the fact that I was a woman. And I'm sure it was felt elsewhere as well – why should this young person and also a female be elected and have an equal say as any male in the Dáil? And at that stage I felt I was disadvantaged on two levels. One, because I was a woman, and two, because I was young.'

De Valera is not alone among the female ministers in being elected to the Dáil at a young age. The former Fianna Fáil Tánaiste Mary Coughlan was 21 when she secured a place on the party's election ticket in 1987. Like de Valera, her youth attracted some attention and a few disparaging remarks: 'Oh, you would hear back, she's far too young, she has no experience, and she will never manage.' Overall though, the feedback Coughlan received was mostly positive, with her gender very much viewed as an advantage: 'A lot of people saw this [election] as very different and thought, Wouldn't it be great that a woman would get elected?' She thinks it set her apart from other contenders: 'It got you out there and got you known because of the fact that you were the only woman.'

Like de Valera, Coughlan also had family political connections. Her election as a Dáil deputy for the Donegal South-West constituency followed two family tragedies. In November 1980, her uncle Clement Coughlan won a seat in a Dáil by-election. During a turbulent political era, Clem contested three general elections in the following two years before being killed in a traffic accident in February 1983. In the subsequent by-election Cathal Coughlan – Clem's brother and Mary's father – retained the seat for Fianna Fáil. Having been a TD for a little over three years, he died suddenly in June 1986. At the time of her father's death, Coughlan was a social sciences student at UCD. Shortly after her father's funeral, she went to Leinster House to collect his belongings. At least, that was the purpose of her visit. For others, it was an opportunity to sound out the young Donegal woman as a potential Fianna Fáil candidate for the 1987 general election: 'The next thing I got a phone call from Mr Haughey to come up to see him. So I would say that was my interview before I even knew it or understood it.' Ultimately a combination of gender and, more importantly, family name played a role in Coughlan's election: 'There's no two ways about it, my father and my uncle's name and reputation for work did carry me hugely.' At the outset of her political career, she says: 'I had a fair majority of people that wanted a Coughlan back. That was really it. They wanted a Coughlan back.'

❧ ❧ ❧

Mary Harney's surname carried no political weight or recognition. When she first ran for the Dáil in 1977, she was a political novice. Fianna Fáil, having lost office in the 1973 election after sixteen years in government, was seeking to promote new candidates, especially women and younger people, to boost its electoral appeal and performance. Against this backdrop, Harney got an unexpected invitation from party officials who came knocking on her door – or rather calling on 'the big public phone' in Trinity College asking, 'Could I speak to Mary Harney?' It was, Harney remembers, Seamus Brennan, 'saying the [Fianna Fáil] national executive have added me [as a candidate] in Dublin South-East. I said to him, "Where is Dublin South-East?" And he said, "Trinity is in Dublin South-East."' Harney was still a student in the college when she contested the general election in 1977.

Like many aspiring female politicians, she had already discovered that getting through the party convention was no easy task. Having been approached by Fianna Fáil while she was a student leader at Trinity and promised a place on the party ticket in Dublin County West, Harney was edged out at the selection convention: 'They said Brian Lenihan will get you through the convention. And of course, he didn't. Liam Lawlor got through instead of me. It is harder for women, there's no doubt, to get through convention. It's probably easier in urban areas, much more difficult in rural areas.'

Harney was eventually added to the party ticket in Dublin South-East, a three-seat constituency in which Fianna Fáil was running three candidates. Harney's parents gave her £40 and the loan of a bicycle. Fianna Fáil paid for accommodation in a house in Sandymount in the heart of the constituency. Peter Gibson, one of her two male running mates, suggested a novel idea to get media and public attention and boost their profiles: 'Peter Gibson, who was a single fella, wanted me to get engaged to him to get publicity. I mean, can you imagine?' Needless to say, no political or romantic match was made for publicity purposes.

With no political connections to guide her, it took the new candidate a little while to become acquainted with practical matters, such as the boundaries of her new constituency. During the campaign, her future colleague in the Progressive Democrats Michael McDowell was a Fine Gael activist: 'He saw me canvassing on the wrong side of the road. It was the other constituency and he didn't tell me. I didn't even know where the constituency was.'

When she was canvassing within her constituency boundaries, Harney was taken aback by the reaction of many female voters: 'You would knock on a door. A woman would answer the door, and she would say, "My husband decides the politics in this house." That was one of the most remarkable things that shocked me as a young woman. She would actually open the door and say, "Hold on, my husband decides the politics." It was just incredible.'

In this period in the late 1970s, Harney remembers that the predominately stay-at-home nature of women's lives was also evident in the profile of both party activists and voters, especially during daytime canvassing: 'An awful lot of canvassing was done during the day, because the women were at home, they weren't out working. The main canvassers would be women during the day, and the main people at home would be women.'

Despite Harney's awkward start on the campaign trail in 1977, she secured a Dáil seat at the second time of asking in Dublin South-West in 1981. Her political CV spanned more than three decades. She contested ten Dáil elections and failed only once, on her first attempt, to take a seat. She also ran successfully in the 1985 local elections and unsuccessfully in the 1989 European Parliament elections. She was first appointed to cabinet in 1997, not just as a government minister but also as the first woman to hold the position of Tánaiste. By any standards this was a significant political career, kick-started without the assistance of being part of a political dynasty. Harney had come a long way from the days of canvassing in the wrong constituency.

In all her election campaigns, Harney says she was helped by women. Her canvassing team was predominantly female: 'Over my career I would say at least 60:40 of the people who canvassed for me were women rather than men, which would be unusual. For the average male candidate, it would be 70:30 [men:women], 80:20 even.'

❖ ❖ ❖

For Mary O'Rourke, there were practical reasons for having female canvassers. O'Rourke, whose political career began in 1974 when she was elected for Fianna Fáil to Athlone Urban District Council, believes women were an asset on the campaign trail.

O'Rourke, who has always been frank in her views says: 'I found them the best canvassers. The guys weren't as thorough in their canvassing.' O'Rourke and her team of female canvassers spent more time on the doorsteps: 'I would go to the door and have the conversation. But the fellas would be, "Come on now, we have to move on, we will never get all the houses done tonight," which was right. I was inclined to be a gabber, I still kind of am a gabber.' O'Rourke's approach challenged conventional canvassing rules: don't waste time and cover as much ground as possible. Despite the time constraints, the approach of O'Rourke and the female members of her team often yielded results while the pragmatism of her male canvassers had its limitations. The women tended to glean more information during these doorstep conversations: 'How many votes are here now? Are there any sons and daughters that are of age for voting? That would be very important. So I noticed they were [more] thorough in their canvassing.'

Several decades later, O'Rourke, now in her eighties, has remained friends with many of the women who knocked on doors for her: 'Some have passed away. And the others, I still often meet them. They went out and they wanted to get me elected. But it wasn't because I was a woman [but] maybe they liked the idea of a woman there.' O'Rourke says many female voters also liked the idea and were supportive of her candidacy: 'Some women might say, "It's nice to have a woman" when they would come to the door.' She always made it her business to speak to both occupants of the house, for practical reasons: 'If a man came to the door, I always said, ask for the woman of the house as well, because we were told this in canvassing. Because they would have two votes, you see.'

Getting voters to open the door in the first place was also a consideration and O'Rourke's party colleague Mary Hanafin states matter of factly that female canvassers were more likely to achieve that outcome: 'People get more and more anxious about opening doors when there are just men outside. We would always pair off a man and a woman, where possible. They [the voters] are more likely to open the door to a woman.' Like O'Rourke, Hanafin is still close to many of the women who canvassed when she was first elected to the Dáil. Hanafin had a mixture of men and women pounding the pavements on her behalf, but she built a core group of women who canvassed for each of her elections: 'I don't know how I started it but I have had my ladies' lunch every single year for the women who canvassed with me since 1997.' That was the year that Hanafin – who eventually served in government – first won a seat for Fianna Fáil.

Hanafin and O'Rourke share much in common. They both attained senior ministerial rank and both had family roots in the political system. Neither saw themselves 'just as a female candidate'. Hanafin's grandfather was a founding member of Fianna Fáil and a local councillor in North Tipperary as was an aunt, while her father, Des, was a long-time member of Seanad Éireann. She grew up 'in a house where men and women equally were able to achieve big office, high office in political life. So I was never aware of a barrier against a woman going forward.'

The same can be said of O'Rourke. Unlike Mary Robinson and Gemma Hussey, who began their political careers in the feminist 1970s, gender politics were not significant for O'Rourke when she entered the political arena: 'There was never any boohoohoo about it.' While acknowledging that Fianna Fáil was a very male party, she says that 'nobody was making a commotion about me being a woman. I was a candidate for Fianna Fáil. That was all that was in it. I never remember saying, gosh, amn't I marvellous, I'm a woman. No.' Her views and experiences are in sharp contrast to many of the other female ministers who sought election in that period, which highlights the differences in their experiences.

O'Rourke was not, however, immune to the negativity that other female politicians faced on the campaign trail at the time. One particular incident stands out for her, when canvassing early one morning on her own. She knocked on a door and a woman with a 'pinny' came out. O'Rourke apologised for the early call, explaining she was trying to do 'little pockets [of canvassing] on her own'. The woman responded, 'I'm so busy myself, what with cooking and cleaning and preparing my children for work, I'm so caught up. I'm so busy.' From her tone, O'Rourke knew instantly that the woman was actually having a go at her: 'I looked her in the eye and I thought, "here goes, ma'am, you looked for this." And I said to her, "Well, I have all that done before I came out this morning. I have two young children. So thank you for meeting me, good morning." And I went off because I knew she never was going to vote for me.' After an unsuccessful run as a Dáil candidate in February 1982, O'Rourke had better luck in the second general election later that same year when she was elected in Longford–Westmeath. She remembers her earlier encounter with the woman with the 'pinny' as very much the exception, not the norm.

❧ ❧ ❧

Many politicians, male and female, start their political careers in local government, which has long been a valuable foothold when running for national office. The time required to build a political career involves huge commitment, always an added challenge when the prospective candidate has family responsibilities. This has been a significant barrier to female participation in political life. Very often, a basic consideration is the actual timing of party and local authority meetings. They are frequently scheduled in the evenings and continue until late in to the night, often ending up in the pub, as Mary Harney recalls. These antisocial hours,

Mary Coughlan says, 'didn't suit women at all'. She remembers attending local meetings in the 1980s that could 'drag on' from 11 a.m. until 6 p.m.

Despite such obstacles, Mary Hanafin says she was never conscious of the small number of female representatives in local politics. Hanafin was elected to Dublin City Council in 1985. Fianna Fáil had 26 of the 52 seats. 'Bertie [Ahern] was leader of the [Fianna Fáil] group [on the council] at the time. He made sure that we all got on committees and groups [depending on] our interests, right. I remember him saying, "OK, Mary, you are a teacher interested in education, you are going on the VEC." He was assigning people responsibilities according to their knowledge and interests.' Gender, according to Hanafin, was not a factor.

Hanafin was fortunate, as other female politicians had different experiences. Jan O'Sullivan – who, like Hanafin and Mary O'Rourke, served as Minister for Education – recalls her tenure in local government. At the time, O'Sullivan was a member of Jim Kemmy's Democratic Socialist Party in Limerick (it merged with Labour in 1990). The party's female members were known as 'Kemmy's Femmies' because of their liberal stance on issues such as family planning services. In 1985, O'Sullivan won a council seat as a Democratic Socialist Party candidate. During her time in the council, she experienced a tendency for 'men to somewhat ignore the opinions of women or, at least, to make their voices louder'. When she was making her contributions at local meetings, she remembers enduring 'constant interruptions' from male colleagues. She says it was more difficult for the views of women to be taken seriously. This led, she thinks, to 'a general sense of solidarity' among the small number of women councillors, irrespective of their political allegiances.

When O'Sullivan was first selected as a Labour candidate in Limerick East in the 1992 general election, she says the transformation of women's role in the party was well advanced: 'There was a time back before I got involved when there were twelve men representing the Labour Party in Leinster House'. O'Sullivan was Kemmy's running mate in the 1992 general election, but despite an uplift in support for Dick Spring's party, she had to wait another six years before becoming a TD.

She was elected in the March 1998 by-election following the death of Jim Kemmy six months earlier. She acknowledges that 'political dynasty' considerations suggested that Joe Kemmy, who was his brother's 'second-in-command', should have the nomination. But she says there was an acknowledgement in Labour of her political track record when Joe Kemmy and other supporters told her: 'Look, you are the one who has done your apprenticeship, you are the one who has been on the council. It's your turn.' She took the seat and retained it in the four subsequent Dáil elections.

❖ ❖ ❖

1992 was a breakthrough year in Irish politics in terms of the number of women elected to the national parliament. There were twenty women in the Dáil, a record number. Just two years earlier, Mary Robinson had been elected Ireland's first female president. The advancement of women in political life seemed to be gathering pace. However, the promise of rapid growth in the early 1990s stalled as the decade progressed. At the subsequent general election in 1997, the number of female TDs stayed at twenty. Nevertheless, 1992 was still a breakthrough of sorts in that a group of women without political connections first entered national politics. Seven of these women went on to serve as senior or junior ministers.

This situation is in sharp contrast to the first generation of female politicians who primarily had family connections to men who had served in the Oireachtas. When Mary Harney first arrived into Leinster House as a new Fianna Fáil senator in 1977, this was still the case. Harney recalls meeting female party colleagues such as Eileen Lemass, whose husband Noel had been a TD and the son of Taoiseach Seán Lemass, and Máire Geoghegan-Quinn and Síle de Valera, both of whom came from political families. The sole female TD from a party that was not Fianna Fáil or Fine Gael in 1977 was Labour's Eileen Desmond, who first won a seat in 1965 left vacant by the death of her husband, Dan, a TD since 1948.

The dynasty dynamic started to change in the early 1980s. 'Garret [FitzGerald, Fine Gael leader] brought the first group of women in 1981, the likes of Nuala Fennell [...] and they didn't come from a political background connected with a man,' Harney recalls. Nora Owen was among that group of new female Fine Gael TDs in 1981: 'Even though I'm a grand-niece of Michael Collins, that wasn't the reason I was elected. We weren't the daughters or the sisters or widows of former TDs. We were elected in our own right. That was a big sea change in 1981.'

This was a trend that was to continue. By the 1992 general election, the majority of the newly elected female TDs, including Niamh Bhreathnach, had, as she puts it, 'no political blood in her at all'. Bhreathnach's trajectory to Leinster House was different to those from political dynasties – or, as she says, 'the wives, the widows and the daughters'. Two other women first elected in 1992 would later become Tánaiste – Labour's Joan Burton (2014–16) and Frances Fitzgerald (2016–17). Harney was the first woman to hold the position, being appointed in 1997 and serving in the role until 2006. Mary Coughlan was Tánaiste from 2008 to 2011. Of these four women, only Coughlan comes from a political family – a sign of changing times.

❖ ❖ ❖

Frances Fitzgerald came to the world of party politics having had a career as a social worker and been a high-profile chairperson of the Council for the Status of Women (now the National Women's Council of Ireland). There were offers from several political parties to run for the Dáil. 'I had a lot of [political] overtures at the time because I was very well-known from the media,' she recalls. She ultimately decided on Fine Gael: 'I had joined the party originally in 1985. [I] had gone along to a local meeting.' She clearly was not impressed by that first meeting because it would be another seven years before she got actively involved in the party. Fitzgerald remembers: 'There was a few people arguing with one another, and I wasn't terribly attracted to it. So I went off. I was very busy with the three kids anyway. I didn't get involved. It's quite hard to get involved in a political party actually. It's still quite hard.'

Before the 1992 general election, former Taoiseach Garret FitzGerald announced his intention to retire from political life, leaving an opening in Dublin South-East. Following an approach from a senior party figure and the former Fine Gael leader himself, Fitzgerald eventually decided to contest the election as a Fine Gael candidate: 'They had polled me. I was polling higher than most other people who they were considering for that constituency.' When she decided to run, she says 'Garret FitzGerald always said to me, "Gosh, it's great that you were a member. I didn't know you were a member."' However, her candidacy met with 'resistance' from some in the local constituency organisation. The row even went public: 'I had a very ugly press release by somebody who was a member at the time, which I found very disturbing.' Her critics, she remembers, were asking: 'Why did [Fine Gael] want to have somebody from outside?' Fierce competition and infighting have always been part and parcel of politics.

Looking back, Fitzgerald wonders, 'if a high-profile man had come in, would that have happened? No, not necessarily. I always think women are a little bit more vulnerable.' At the selection convention in Dublin South-East, Fitzgerald along with the sitting TD, Joe Doyle, were chosen to run for Fine Gael. She got elected but Doyle lost out: 'While I was delighted to be elected, the constituency were disappointed there weren't still two seats. And of course, it shows the absolute competitive nature of politics, the ups and downs.' It also shows how cruel politics can be, to both men and women.

❧ ❧ ❧

Political parties are pragmatic if not always principled in their electoral strategies. By 2011, female candidates were being sought by most of the main political parties to run in the general election but the approach lacked consistency and progress was still slow. While it was the exception and not the norm for voters to be faced with an all-male line-up on their ballot papers in 2011, just 15 per cent of the candidates that stood for election were women. Numerically, there were more female candidates than in 2007, but the total number had only increased by four and the percentage of female candidates had actually decreased by 2.2 per cent since 2007.[25] Heather Humphreys and Regina Doherty, both of whom later attained senior ministerial positions, were first elected as Fine Gael TDs in 2011. For both women, the decision to stand for election was, in part, due to timing. However, even though they were headhunted by Fine Gael party officials, they still had to endure the rough-and-tumble of election campaigns.

Humphreys was managing a credit union in Co. Cavan when Fine Gael approached her about running in the 2004 local elections. With the end of the dual mandate, which allowed Oireachtas members to also sit on local councils, in 2003, Fine Gael had a vacancy on Monaghan County Council. Humphreys had not been a member of any political party prior to 2003. She recalls being approached one Sunday evening and by 2 p.m. the following afternoon, she had accepted the offer: 'I thought, this is an opportunity. I said, yeah, I will go for it. And the main reason being, I felt I would have been compromising myself to some extent in terms of giving out about something or saying things should be changed.' She was co-opted onto the council and subsequently won the seat in her own right in the local elections the following year.

Humphreys feels she was fortunate: 'I just happened to be in the right place at the right time.' A number of other people, including her brother, were considered for the council vacancy before Fine Gael came to her door: 'They had been around a few, I'm not under any illusion here. I wasn't the first person they asked.' She attributes the approach made to her to the party 'looking for women'. When it came to the 2011 general election, Humphreys was one of four Fine Gael candidates on the party ticket in the five-seat Cavan–Monaghan constituency. She says the campaign was 'a tough fight' but that she 'wasn't treated differently in any way, or I didn't get any special favours being a woman. It was dog eat dog.' Ironically this probably demonstrates that the Fine Gael politician was treated the same as other candidates.

She took the final seat of the three that Fine Gael won in Cavan–Monaghan on what was an exceptional day for the party locally and nationally. Humphreys was a surprising choice when she was elevated from the Fine Gael backbenches in a cabinet reshuffle in 2014 to become the Minister for the Arts, Heritage and the Gaeltacht. 'My mother always said there's no job that a woman can't do,' she recalls.

Like Humphreys, Doherty was not Fine Gael's first choice as a candidate at the 2007 general election. As she recalls, the preferred candidate for Meath East withdrew upon becoming pregnant. She also attributes her selection to the party wanting a woman on the ticket. With the sitting TD Shane McEntee situated in the northern part of the constituency, Fine Gael was 'looking for a woman' in Doherty's area. When she was first approached to run, she 'was pregnant on number four but I had two boys at the time, both of whom had special needs.'

Doherty had to make a decision. One factor that motivated her was the allocation of resources for children. At the time, Doherty had been actively involved in campaigns to change policy in this area but felt it was like 'banging your head off a brick wall'. Over Christmas dinner, her mother influenced her decision to seek the nomination, arguing: '"You would have better luck if you were on the inside." And that was the reason that actually made me change my mind.'

Her mother was no stranger to politics. She had run as a Fine Gael candidate in the local elections in 1979. She was unsuccessful but remained active in party politics. For Regina Doherty, this meant accompanying her parents to party events. She recalls attending a Fine Gael Ard Fheis in her communion dress, but she was not complaining as it proved beneficial: 'I made a good few bob', she says. She also collected autographs from party figures, including Garret FitzGerald and John Bruton: 'I have a little autograph book at home with all of the names of the people who wrote, "To Regina" and "Sweet little Regina".'

As she began her political career, Doherty faced attitudes that were not dissimilar to those experienced almost thirty years earlier by women like Máire Geoghegan-Quinn and Nora Owen. When she first ran for the party's nomination, some comments were made about her being seven months pregnant. There was a view that 'I should be at home minding my kids as opposed to thinking or considering at this stage of my life a career in politics.' Doherty had, however, weighed up the implications of what becoming a TD would mean for her family life. When she was first approached to run in the 2007 general election, she thought, '"Are you all mad as brushes?" But obviously the idea sprung a little seed in my head and then I decided, "Sure, what harm can it do?"' At the time, Doherty was a relative unknown: 'Our [selection] convention was in May. Kate was born in August, and in September I took time off work and started canvassing. Nobody had a ball's notion who I was. I started canvassing a couple of hours a day, every single day, which was painful. Because you would go to the door, you would have to explain to them, "Excuse me, my name is …" and you would have to go into the whole spiel of who you are, where you came from and why you were even there.'

Doherty was unsuccessful in 2007 but took a seat in 2011, which she retained five years later. She was appointed Minister for Employment Affairs and Social Protection in 2017. As a relatively new female politician, Doherty has seen how the role of women in party politics has changed in recent times: 'There's an awful lot more men in Fine Gael than there are women. And actually, an awful lot of the women members are the wives of the men who come to the meetings. So I would have a lot of men canvassing. It has changed over the years. I have a canvass team that goes out every Friday. I would say now we are about half women, half men, where we wouldn't have been in the beginning.'

❧ ❧ ❧

After the 2016 general election, the number of female TDs surpassed the 30 mark for the first time. Both Fine Gael and

Fianna Fáil found it a real challenge to reach the 30 per cent gender-quota target for female candidates in 2016. In the end, all the political parties met the quota requirements, but in some cases, proactive measures had to be taken. For example, constituency organisations were sometimes instructed to ensure a female candidate came through a selection convention. This ensured eleven more women were candidates in 2016 than would otherwise be the case. Some female candidates were also added to the ticket after selection conventions. Of the 33 candidates added to those already selected at local conventions, nineteen (almost 60 per cent) were women.[26]

Josepha Madigan, who contested her first general election in Dublin–Rathdown in 2016, states, 'I was a gender-quota candidate.' She has mixed views about it: 'I felt that I had a lot more to prove in a sense, because you don't want to be just on a ticket because you are a woman.' In 2016 Fine Gael suffered a serious electoral defeat, dropping from 76 to 50 seats on the 2011 General Election, so being on the ballot paper was no guarantee of election. Her party colleague former minister Alan Shatter failed to get elected and Madigan won the only Fine Gael seat in the constituency: 'I like to think that I have proved myself since then in terms of my capabilities rather than people perceiving me just as a female who got on the ticket because she's female.'

Madigan's entry into national politics owes much to an approach from Olivia Mitchell, a former Fine Gael TD for Dublin South. Mitchell asked if she would run in the 2014 local elections: 'I remember when she said it to me, I looked behind me to see was she talking to somebody else.' Madigan's father, who died in 2014, had been a long-time local councillor, first with Fianna Fáil and later as an Independent. But despite this family association, she says a career in politics 'genuinely hadn't crossed my mind' as she progressed her legal career. In the aftermath of the economic collapse, she canvassed for Olivia Mitchell in the 2011 general election: 'And then I joined a branch. And then I joined the constituency. And then I became a local election candidate and then a general election candidate. But it was never a plan.' And then she became a minister – not even two years had passed since she was first elected.

There are numerous reasons for Madigan's victory. The introduction of gender quotas simply, but critically, ensured she was a Fine Gael candidate. Now Madigan holds the historic distinction of officially being Ireland's first gender-quota candidate to be appointed to cabinet and the 19th Irish woman to serve as a senior minister.

2

LEINSTER HOUSE – THE
CORRIDORS OF POWER

*The first thing that struck me when I went into
Leinster House was how old everybody seemed. Like, I
was 24. I just thought, 'Oh my God, I will be gone out
of here before I'm 40. I thought they were just so old.'*

MARY HARNEY

Mary Harney vividly recalls her first impressions of
Leinster House following her appointment to the
Seanad in 1977. Despite planning to leave after sixteen
years, her career plans clearly changed: by the time she bowed
out of national politics in 2011, her time in Leinster House had
spanned 34 years. She has the distinction of being the longest-
serving female TD in the history of the state.

Harney's recollections of the home of the national parliament
during the late 1970s and 1980s are not very positive. The building,
as she recalls, was populated by 'elderly males … [and it] was not
a very friendly place for women.' The absence of women was not
just visible in the Dáil chamber. The ranks of other professions in
Leinster House – specifically, the political correspondents and the
ushers – were predominately male. Women were a rare species.

'It wasn't a place where you saw many women,' Harney recalls and neither she nor Mary Coughlan can remember when they first saw a female usher working there. In fact, the first female usher arrived in Leinster House in 1994, some seventeen years after Harney's career as a national politician began. It was a highly gendered workplace, with women over-represented only among the secretarial staff. Síle de Valera remembers sitting in the Dáil chamber at the time and looking up to the parliamentary press gallery, where there were very few female faces. 'Both the Dáil chamber and those covering the stories reflected the community at the time, where women unfortunately hadn't a big say in society,' de Valera recalls.

Leinster House was an overwhelmingly male workplace up to the 1990s. Many of the women who served as senior ministers point to the prevailing atmosphere and culture, the lack of facilities for women and the level of scrutiny they were subjected to as members of a minority. For most women, it was not a welcoming or encouraging workplace. On some occasions though, being one of the handful of female politicians in national political life brought a small advantage. After the 1981 general election, Nora Owen was one of five new female Fine Gael TDs. Their arrival meant the number of women in the Dáil had reached double digits – eleven out of 166 TDs – for the first time. Shortly after her election, Owen was walking into Leinster House with her party colleague Seán Barrett when they met the late Brian Farrell, one of the main current affairs presenters on RTÉ: 'We walked in the door and Brian came in after us, and said to Seán, "Seán, will you come out to do an interview?"' Farrell proceeded to put his hand on Owen's hand as he apologised, 'I hope you don't mind me borrowing your husband, I just want to do an interview with him'. There was some laughter before Owen replied, 'Well, first of all, he's not my husband, and secondly, I'm a TD as well.' She introduced herself to a 'very embarrassed' Brian Farrell. The broadcaster, recovered quickly: 'He pushed Seán to one side and took me out and interviewed me.' It was an early example for Owen of how the media tended to give attention to the small number of female politicians. 'If you spoke in the Dáil you got quoted, whereas fifteen men might have spoken and only two of them were quoted. You kind of stood out because you were the smaller number,' she says.

There were, however, some very practical disadvantages of this minority status for female politicians in the 1970s and 1980s. Mary Coughlan describes the facilities for women as 'chronic'. There was a particular problem with toilet facilities. In some parts of Leinster House, the location of the toilets reflected the position of women in Irish politics at the time: on the periphery. Recalling the day she first arrived in Leinster House, Máire Geoghegan-Quinn says, 'I think I spent a day asking people, where's the ladies'? [...] and an awful lot of the men didn't know where it was because it was kind of tucked away in a little corner.' In many areas of the building, Coughlan recalls that the female toilets were 'as far away now as a lighthouse'. This could be problematic, as Owen remembers. She was asked to second the nomination of Fine Gael leader Garret FitzGerald as Taoiseach in December 1982: 'You know they ring the bells and, of course, I was so nervous having to stand up and do this,' she says. Before the vote, Owen recalls asking an usher in one part of the building where the ladies' toilets were. The Fine Gael TD feared she would end up missing the start of the Dáil proceedings – and her high-profile role in the nomination of her party leader as Taoiseach. As she made her way to the Dáil chamber, she was 'terrified I had got locked out'.

In the private members' bar, there was no ladies' toilet. Like most of the facilities in Leinster House, they had been planned for men. Owen recalls that, 'inside the door of the members' bar, there was a men's toilet. We [women] had to go the whole way out into the corridor to a public toilet outside the visitors' bar.' Of the overall lavatory situation, Harney pointedly notes that 'the men's was always closer to the action than the ladies".

The handful of female politicians in the 1970s did have access to a dedicated room in Leinster House known as 'the women's room'. This small room had a leather couch, a desk with some chairs and a telephone. 'It was a tiny room,' Harney says. 'My memory of going in there was that Kit Ahern would be in there, and Eileen Desmond and Eileen Lemass. And they would be all sitting there, just chatting and there was one phone. You would just hang out. You could be sitting there for hours.' Geoghegan-Quinn also recalls the women's room but can't remember ever using it: 'I did feel there was a need for people to meet and have a chat in an informal setting rather than going to the bar or restaurant, but I didn't think it should be confined to women.'

For those female politicians who were uncomfortable going into the Dáil bar for a coffee or a drink, the 'women's room' had an additional attraction. 'In my early years when they had the women's room, I rarely went into the members' bar. It just wasn't a thing you did,' Harney recalls, adding that 'it wasn't seen as a place for women. It was probably a bit of a hangover from the pubs that didn't allow women in. That probably spilled into Leinster House for far too long.' The net result, according to Harney, was that the member's bar 'wasn't a place for women. It wasn't a place that was friendly towards women. You were conscious that you were in a male place.' Some of the other female politicians had similar feelings and avoided the bar. Mary Robinson was not a frequent visitor: 'I would go into the bar with people. I would never go in on my own. And it would only be on rare, rare enough occasions.' It was 'a very male place', she remembers.

It is a sign of the prejudices of that era that many female politicians, who were no means pushovers or shrinking violets, felt uncomfortable and sometimes intimidated going into the bar. Nora Owen, who would later serve as Minister for Justice, was one of them. She says the members' bar was sometimes even 'more intimidating than going into the chamber'. The new Fine Gael women TDs elected in 1981 would meet in the bar for coffee early in the day or sometimes for a drink when the Dáil was sitting late in the evening: 'We did look for support when we went in because it was very male. You see, the men had got used to being in there and there were one or two – I won't give names – who [would say] "What are you bitches talking about? What are you women talking about?" I don't know whether they ever said "bitches". They would be kind of goading us. Nobody ever said, "What are you fellas talking about?"'

Gemma Hussey had similar experiences in the members' bar: 'If they saw two or three women sitting together, they would say, "What's this plotting going on? There's some terrible plotting going on." They would forget that they were always together, the gangs of men. But if they saw two or three women together, [they would ask] "What are you doing?"' Change came slowly during the 1980s, as Owen recalls: 'You had to learn to say "None of your business, what are you talking about?" You had to learn how to answer back. And there were some of the rural deputies, including one of ours, I remember, that were sometimes quite unpleasant. And you kind of felt, well, do I have the right to be in here?' Looking back, Owen regrets not been more assertive in dealing with these chauvinistic attitudes: 'We probably should have been more robust in telling them, "Look, I'm elected the same as you, now just shut up and go back to your group."'

Frances Fitzgerald was another politician who generally avoided the members' bar following her election as a Fine Gael

TD in 1992. She never felt intimidated but simply was not a fan of the drinking culture at the time. 'It was a place where the guys went,' she says, especially TDs from outside Dublin, for whom it 'was very much almost home from home, it was their social place. And it was mostly men. You didn't find that many women going in there at that time.'

According to Fitzgerald, today the bar and restaurant are 'much more social in terms of people having their lunch in there all the time. It is a space where politicians meet.' Some habits, however, remain: 'You stick with your own party mostly. [The restaurant] is still quite segregated, which I always think is very funny. That even when Fine Gael got more people elected, we still ended up in the same tables, even though they were smaller than the tables that Fianna Fáil have on the right-hand side.' Former Labour leader Joan Burton also believes the members' bar has changed significantly in more recent times: 'You could ban alcohol in the Dáil bar tomorrow, provided you kept the tea and coffee arrangements. I, for one, would not care and I would imagine that about 80 per cent of the House would feel like that.' Nowadays, Burton says the bar is more akin to a tea and coffee shop for members with a very small number drinking alcohol there in the evenings.

In the past, there was also an expectation about how women were expected to act and speak in Leinster House – with what was considered un-ladylike behaviour noted. Geoghegan-Quinn recalls socialising with some Fianna Fáil party colleagues after the 1977 general election. 'I remember using the f-word in the restaurant or in the bar. And that came about because I was in company of people who were using it in the conversation. And P[ádraig] Flynn, of all people, [said] "Now, Madam," he said to me, looking across at me, "I'm going to charge you 50 pence every time you use the f-word in future." Jesus, by the end of the first week he had a pile in the jar, and he did, he followed through on it. And it cured me.' It would be interesting to find out how many of her male colleagues were also subjected to this exercise. Labour's Jan O'Sullivan says, 'People apologise to me all the time for using bad language. And I think that's ridiculous.' She admits to using such language 'occasionally', prompting shocked reactions: 'They kind of look at me and say, "I never thought you would use that word." So maybe that is sexist in a way.'

Many of the women who attained senior ministries believe that the 'macho culture' that permeated Leinster House in the past has been somewhat diluted but not completely eradicated, due to the recent election of more female politicians. Today, just over 20 per cent of TDs are women, still low by international standards but an increase nevertheless on previously very low numbers. With this improving gender profile, O'Sullivan feels Leinster House has changed: 'The kinds of things that were talked about in conversation in the Dáil bar, the members' bar, was stuff that women weren't particularly interested in talking about. The number of women in here has changed it. I think numbers are really important. We are still obviously in a minority but I think [in] this Dáil there is more of a feeling of women around the place. I think gradually the fact that the numbers of women have increased has made a difference to the atmosphere around here.'

Gemma Hussey, who was first elected to the Dáil in February 1982, felt the absence of female colleagues. Sometimes, she says, 'you would love to sit down with a woman, you know. If you were stuck in the place late at night and you would love to sit down and throw off your shoes and talk to a woman.' The divide between the world of the dominant male politicians and the small number of female TDs in the early 1980s was evident in a variety of different ways. Hussey recalls 'an awful lot of watching of football matches on the televisions in Leinster House. There would be crowds of men shouting and roaring at the television.'

Frances Fitzgerald recalls the culture shock when she visited Leinster House even before she became a TD: 'I remember being astounded at the number of men and the male atmosphere. It was like another world to what I had been exposed to, compared to the world of equality. It seemed like a throwback.' There were further shocks for Fitzgerald when she became a TD in 1992. She noticed the number of men eating 'fries in the morning' in the Dáil restaurant. '[Leinster House] had a very male traditional feel about it. There were a lot of older men as well. There weren't that many younger women. I mean, I was 42. I was probably one of the younger ones.' At that time, Fitzgerald was a Fine Gael backbench TD, conscious that she was part of the minority in a working environment defined by 'male interests': 'I think the secretaries were regarded in a certain way as well. You know, they were very much the handmaidens to the men. That was the model – [despite the fact that] they were doing so much work behind the scenes.' For her part, Nora Owen remembers 'a lot of laddishness' and rude jokes: 'If it was too rude, I said, "Oh for goodness sake, don't be telling that".' According to Geoghegan-Quinn, these experiences were illustrative of the existence of 'a bit of a macho culture'.

❧ ❧ ❧

Leinster House did not stand in isolation from wider Irish society. Notwithstanding the encouragement Mary Coughlan received from many quarters when she embarked on her political career, she says the Dáil 'reflected a lot of the society that I represented in Donegal, in that the party [Fianna Fáil] would have been made up of older people, older men, who would have absolutely no time for women or young people.'

A number of the female ministers elected before the turn of century say they were, by and large, left to find their own way in a work environment dominated by men. Most were struck by the lack of general supports available to new TDs. Máire Geoghegan-Quinn says when she was first elected in 1975, 'there was no such thing as the whip or the chairman of the party or anybody being appointed to say to new people, "this is where the post office is, this is where your office is going to be, this is where you get supplies for your office, this is going to be your secretary". You know, like would happen in any other job.'

On being appointed to the Seanad as a Taoiseach's nominee in 1977, Mary Harney had a similar experience of being 'on your own, learning the ropes'. She says, 'I am involved in a lot of corporations now, you get an induction programme, you get a big file with all the details. That didn't happen.' Mary Coughlan recognises the sense of isolation experienced by new TDs but admits she had the advantage of coming from a political background with family members who had served in the Oireachtas: 'My uncle's secretary became my father's secretary, and she was my secretary for a long time. So there was that continuity within the office, which was hugely important. I feel sorry for somebody who is coming in green into the Oireachtas, with absolutely no experience of how to do anything.' This also applied to new male members of the Oireachtas.

To overcome such challenges, the support of long-standing TDs was sometimes necessary when navigating Leinster House. Party allegiances did not matter. Joan Burton recalls on her first day as a new Labour TD in 1992, Fianna Fáil's Mary O'Rourke came up to her in the restaurant and offered to show her around the building. Burton says, 'Your first day in the Dáil is like being back in primary school. It seems like an awfully big place with an awful lot of people who know what they are doing and you don't know anything.' In terms of becoming acquainted with Leinster House, Mary Mitchell O'Connor, who was elected for Fine Gael in 2011, famously drove her car over the plinth outside Leinster House: 'It was completely silly of me. I look back now and I think, "How did I do that?" It was embarrassing. But you know, things happen.' Mitchell O'Connor was most unfortunate that the incident was caught on camera.

Overall, the facilities and supports for new TDs have improved dramatically since the 1970s and 1980s, not just in terms of offices and back-up staff but also the general work environment in Leinster House and the buildings in the vicinity of Kildare Street where many of the female ministers have their offices. The increased number of female politicians has forced the creation of a more gender-neutral workplace, although many features of a long-time male-dominated world remain, as illustrated in the stories that follow.

❧ ❧ ❧

Forty years on from the experiences of politicians like Mary Harney, Máire Geoghegan-Quinn and Síle de Valera, Jan O'Sullivan remains conscious that female TDs are still a minority and account for only one in five members of the Dáil. 'I think that sends out a message, particularly to the schoolchildren that you see up in the [public] gallery,' the Labour TD says.

Others have a different perspective. Both Heather Humphreys and Regina Doherty were elected as new Fine Gael TDs in the 2011 general election. They also noticed the large number of male faces in Leinster House although neither woman was overly concerned by this reality when entering the building for the first time. 'This was the way it was. Obviously, a lot more men had been elected than women. But that's the decision of the electorate,' Humphreys says. Doherty is conscious of the gender imbalance but she says, 'You don't get up every morning and think, "I'm a woman, and I'm going to work as a woman." You just get up and you go to work.' She recalls a meeting of the new Fine Gael parliamentary party after the 2011 general election: 'And sure, typical fashion, I was late. I arrived into the back of the Mansion House room, and all I saw was grey suits and bald heads. Now maybe that says more about the people that we have in Fine Gael. But the vast majority of people in the room were men in grey suits with thinning hair.' Reflecting on what needs to change, Doherty agrees with O'Sullivan: 'Young women need to see examples of what they can be when they grow up.'

Katherine Zappone strongly agrees. She was first elected at the 2016 general election, in which the highest number of female TDs was elected since the foundation of the state. An Independent TD, who was appointed to cabinet on arriving in the Dáil, Zappone is mindful of the under-representation of female politicians in the national parliament: 'I'm never unconscious of the fact that I am a woman, and I have mostly male colleagues. And I still feel that way.' She is also conscious of being in another minority: 'I was the first to be openly lesbian, to use the word lesbian, and I still use that word rather than gay, which is inclusive of everything, because I still think gay is a male-identified word.' Zappone remembers when she first mentioned her sexuality in the Seanad, of which she was a member from 2011 to 2016: 'I would have used it a couple of times and I do think that my colleagues, women or men, but especially the men, would have been uncomfortable hearing that.' But, she says, 'when I used it the third or fourth time, people weren't uncomfortable anymore. And when I talked about being a married lesbian, even before it was accepted here, that was really important to me.'

It is understandable that Zappone would be conscious of the response that she received in the Seanad as to what was a significant personal and public declaration. For others, simply speaking in the Dáil chamber has been challenging, with many of the female ministers highlighting what they see as the prevailing gendered culture in terms of the atmosphere and the discourse.

Former TDs recall being self-conscious in the chamber, especially as there were so few women. Being in a minority impacted on Nora Owen's perception of her role as a TD when she first took a seat in 1981: 'You would be afraid to heckle. You would see some of the others heckling, and you would be saying to yourself, "Oh God, I daren't." You would be a bit nervous because the media were all up in the gallery. And you wouldn't want to make a fool of yourself. So you tended to stay kind of quiet.' Some would argue that such restraint in heckling may not have been such a bad thing. But this most likely demonstrates a lack of confidence, which Owen overcame the longer she served as a TD: 'I became a good heckler, in my own time. But I tended to try and stay fairly self-effacing.'

Almost a decade after Owen was first elected, Niamh Bhreathnach was returned as a Labour TD in Dún Laoghaire in 1992. She found the chamber 'a bear pit': 'You walk down those steps. It's very challenging.' Frances Fitzgerald was also conscious of the atmosphere in the Dáil chamber when she was first elected: 'It's so gladiatorial and so hierarchical.' Mary Hanafin agrees: 'The Dáil is very big, very formal, very adversarial. I think an outsider looking in sees a very adversarial system, sees a lot of aggression, and they don't want to be a part of it.' This adversarial nature was something that Mary Harney also found off-putting in a Dáil career stretching from 1981 to 2011: 'My view is that women in general are more interested in the issues and less interested in the politics. Men are the reverse, very often. So I often found some of what passes for politics on the floor of the Dáil disillusioning, to be honest. It was more about the game than it was about the issue. A lot of macho performances.'

- Síle de Valera's experience of the Dáil chamber was also of a place that was 'very confrontational' and 'very macho'. In a political career that included representing constituencies in Dublin and Clare, and serving in cabinet from 1997 to 2002, de Valera found many colleagues 'would never admit to being wrong' and would never admit to 'another party even having the semblance of a good idea'. There was a different approach, she recalls, at Oireachtas committees, especially on the women's committee where TDs were 'very pragmatic'. She says politicians would 'listen to each other, and if there was a good idea, they would agree and get on with it. In other words, a practical approach to work.'

Ultimately, the adversarial approach in the Dáil puts both women and men off becoming involved in politics, according to Mary Coughlan: 'It would put most people off at the best of times. But I think it would put women off, because that's not the way women behave to each other, you know, in my view.' Coughlan believes not having a thin skin is essential to career progression in politics. But she argues that 'there's a cut and thrust and then there's a fine line. And sometimes it goes over the fine line when people are personal and pass-remarkable.' Having arrived at the cabinet table in 2002, Coughlan was appointed Minister for Enterprise, Trade and Employment six years later – at the outset of the economic crisis. Leo Varadkar was her Fine Gael counterpart on the opposition benches. Coughlan took exception to Varadkar comparing her to Sarah Palin, the gaffe-prone 2008 Republican vice-presidential candidate in the United States. 'It wasn't fair, because he had absolutely no idea the hell that I went through in that department. I wouldn't say he [Varadkar] is sexist, to be fair to him. But it was just a nice, easy, cheap shot. And that's a party thing.'

According to the female ministers, party politics is generally non-discriminatory, with most opponents caring little for the gender of their sparring partners who are targeted in an equal and often brutal fashion. However, some of them feel their contributions often attract more scrutiny and carry less weight. Joan Burton says that if she was a painter she 'could paint a picture of all the sighing, muttering and rolling of eyes' by men who are saying, '"Now what is she going on about?" And that's not just me. That's about all the different "shes" in Leinster House.' She believes it has taken 'a long period for people in Leinster House to really accept women as equals'. As a result, Burton argues, women have to be 'quite resilient and pushy enough' to show that they are not 'some kind of add-on or decoration'. Surviving the Dáil chamber, Burton says, requires 'sharp elbows and being prepared to just take it on'. She feels, however, that the very combative nature of the chamber remains a 'major deterrent in younger women saying, "I would go into politics"'.

While many of the female ministers feel that this adversarial approach cuts across both genders, Burton, who first won a Dáil seat in Dublin West in 1992, believes that 'it is much more difficult for women to respond with a really strong vigour. And it is much easier for men to put the boot in on the perceived inadequacies of women.' She says, 'It's a syndrome that I often call "too tall, too small, too fat, too thin" and so on. In other words, for men to be in politics they just have to be average plus; for women to be successful in politics, they in effect have to have elements of superwomen.'

Frances Fitzgerald highlights the physical layout of the Dáil chamber as worthy of change to ease the combative nature of political engagement: 'Even the way it's tiered down. You go into the Swedish parliament, it's all just on the same level. You know, I don't think it's necessarily the best way to do business. I think we have a lot of improvements to make.' However, Fitzgerald believes that 'the Dáil is the Dáil' and that male and female politicians are treated equally in the chamber: 'If they can go for you, they will go for you.' In her experience, opponents did not treat her differently because she is a woman: 'I think it's more or less the same. There might be a bit more identification male-to-male from time to time than there is male-to-female.'

Having been elected in 2011 in one of the most recent intake of female TDs, Mary Mitchell O'Connor's assessment of how business is done in the Dáil chamber does not differ greatly from that of the female politicians who held seats decades earlier: 'I will put an inverted-commas around the "gentlemen" who regularly shout and roar. And often what they will do is, they will come into the chamber once a week. They will shout and roar, and then they are usually gone before the minister or the Taoiseach even gets to answer the question.' Anyone who has spent time watching debates in the Dáil would accept that such behaviour is not confined to the opposition benches. Party politics aside, Mitchell O'Connor believes the under-representation of women in Irish political life is a contributing factor: 'It is laddy. The behaviour is macho. It's aggressive. It's very off-putting.' She argues that any check of the Dáil record would show that female politicians generally work differently: 'Women are able to do the business in a quiet way. That's their modus operandi.'

Jan O'Sullivan puts the difference in approach between men and women in the Dáil chamber down to the fact women are not as good at 'playing to the gallery': 'I think women generally don't do that, women generally say what they mean.' Josepha Madigan, first elected for Fine Gael in 2016 and appointed to cabinet at the end of 2017, believes it is really important that female politicians 'stay feminine and that we don't become masculine to get our point across. I think sometimes as women we come across too abrasive because we are trying to be into that, you know, masculine strand, when in fact femininity is a strength in itself.'

Many of the female ministers who highlight the under-representation of women as influencing the atmosphere in the Dáil and the behaviour of some TDs in the chamber also note that disruptive behaviour is not exclusive to one gender. Heather Humphreys believes that some of her colleagues 'put on an act, and that brings publicity' and that 'there's some women good at it too'. Regina Doherty admits that female politicians 'are well able to have a good old row and a ding-dong … [but that] what you are probably less likely to see [with women] is the jeering and the bipartisanship'. Katherine Zappone agrees that women can also be 'culprits', but there are 'more men'. She is also not sure if this behaviour is 'just the Irish culture of politics'.

❧ ❧ ❧

One dynamic that transcends Irish politics is the tendency to label female politicians. In her recent autobiography, *What Happened*, former United States presidential candidate Hillary Clinton addressed the way in which female politicians are negatively tagged as 'shrill' or 'domineering' when their male counterparts are considered 'emphatic' and 'powerful'. Clinton argues that this has a damaging impact on public perceptions of female politicians. Many of the women who served as senior ministers are more than familiar with this trend and the danger of being stereotyped as 'bossy', 'screeching' and 'hysterical'. These terms are not confined to the political sphere. 'Bossy? Yeah, I often used to hear that comment,' Mary O'Rourke admits. 'I had been a teacher. And people are inclined to think teachers are bossy. I remember a couple of times people saying, "Oh, don't be giving us that old teacher-talk now" or "Don't be doing the bossy teacher on us"'. Her male colleagues who arrived into the world of politics from the teaching profession rarely received these types of comment: 'Oh, not at all. No.' When Mary Hanafin was first elevated to cabinet, she recalls being described as 'a schoolmarm' due to her teaching background: 'They are probably saying, "Don't be treating us like children." But it was because you were a teacher rather than because you were a woman.'

In her experience as a two-term TD and a former cabinet minister, Mary Mitchell O'Connor believes national politics is 'a difficult space' for women: 'It's difficult to be yourself. Is your voice too soft? Is it too loud? You know, you have to try and get it just right.' Heather Humphreys says women can be labelled 'pushy' while their male counterparts are seen as 'assertive'. She believes that 'women have to be very careful, because nobody listens to a screeching woman.' She adds, 'I am conscious that you have to keep the tone of your voice down. Because once you hear somebody screeching, and I hate to say it but if you hear a screeching woman, you switch off, you don't listen. [Men have] a deeper voice. And they are not as inclined to hit the high decibels that women do.'

This view is not shared by Jan O'Sullivan, who believes most women 'don't shout' but rather 'speak in a fairly measured way'. She also believes that female politicians 'by and large tend to listen to each other, and listen to others, whereas men tend to want to get their point of view across more.'

'Your voice is never right,' Joan Burton says. The former Labour leader, who has attracted her share of negative commentary, asserts: 'It's too strong or it's too weak. It's too sweet or it's too sharp. I think you have to get over that [because] where are the perfect men that at any stage have inhabited our Dáil?' Her Labour colleague Jan O'Sullivan identifies Burton and the

Sinn Féin president Mary Lou McDonald as female politicians who are often considered 'too strident'. But, O'Sullivan argues, if a male politician spoke in a similar manner, he would be 'considered to be strong'. O'Sullivan thinks there is a double standard at play: 'I have heard comments about the interaction between Mary Lou and Joan [in the Dáil]. If two men were engaging like that, it would be barely noticed. I think it is sexist.'

The exchanges between Burton and McDonald that O'Sullivan is referencing took place when Burton was Tánaiste from 2014 to 2016 in the latter half of the term of the Fine Gael–Labour coalition. Burton feels there was 'a lot of stereotyping' in the commentary around their exchanges, but that the debate was led by politics, not personality: 'I don't recall ever saying anything personal about her and I don't recall her ever saying anything personal about me, either in terms of let's say appearance or voice or, you know, just kind of slaying the individual as a person. I don't think either of us ever did that. We debated the issues hot and heavy. We debated approaches and facts.'

Mary Harney notes that the double standards in how female politicians are treated is not a uniquely Irish phenomenon: 'If you take Margaret Thatcher, she was regarded as a man. I know it sounds like a contradiction, but that is a fact. Because she was tough and was all the things that people feel women shouldn't be. And then if you are on the other extreme, and you are emotional and sensitive and weepy, you are finished.' She is of the firm view that 'if you are the kind of person that cries easily, [politics is] not the place to be'.

Many of the female ministers agree with this point about displaying emotions. Mary O'Rourke admits she was conscious of not showing emotions in public: 'Yes, I was. I don't know why that was. Maybe because I didn't want to be the whingeing woman or the crying woman.' Mary Coughlan says showing emotion 'wouldn't have been seen as being professional. [You'd get the] "that's women for you" type of comment.' Coughlan admits that even when under pressure she worked hard not to show anger: 'It didn't matter what they said to me, if they kicked me around the room and if everybody ate me alive, I was going to stick it out.'

Gemma Hussey says her only difficulty around an all-male cabinet table was maintaining her composure: 'Women are emotional. I'm emotional. At times, we would have been at the cabinet table for maybe five hours with a short break. Garret was not known for short cabinet meetings. And the next thing they were going to cut my budget again. And I would sometimes feel emotional. And I would sometimes feel that I might weep.' Hussey, however, says she always resisted the urge to shed a tear: 'I was aware that that was simply not on as a woman.' She recalls being left 'grievously disappointed' after the cabinet reshuffle in 1986 saw her moved from Education to Social Welfare. While she later cried in private with her husband, she had actually experienced an emotional (Taoiseach) Garret FitzGerald when news of her ministerial move was confirmed: 'He kept saying that he was worried I would lose my seat because the teachers were all ganging up against me. I said, "Please don't worry about that." Garret was in tears, put his arms around me and said, "That's a wonderful thing to say."'

As Minister for Justice, Nora Owen says she 'had to be careful, because if it was a case about a child or a woman or domestic violence, it was quite easy to find yourself filling up. I think you knew you shouldn't blubber.' Owen did allow her emotions to show when she lost her seat in the 2002 general election. The moment was captured by the cameras and became one of the talking points of the election. One of the reasons it attracted so much attention was because the Dublin North constituency was one of those selected for a trial of electronic voting technology.

With no tallies available in the constituency, there was no advance warning of the likely outcome. Owen was on the platform with the other candidates when the results were announced: 'I didn't mind that there was an emotion, that it looked like an emotional thing. I think it was important that people saw it was upsetting. And it is upsetting. It's like a bereavement.'

One of most memorable moments of Mary Robinson's presidency was also captured on television, when she responded emotionally to what she had encountered after visiting famine-stricken Somalia. Robinson, however, felt uncomfortable afterwards: 'I think the training of a barrister is to take cases for people and to be their advocate but not to show emotion.' The former president adds, 'When I did find myself breaking down a little bit with the press in Kenya, following the visit to Somalia, I was furious with myself. Because I was not doing professionally what I should be doing. I was showing weakness, you know. That was my kind of training.' She has changed since leaving Áras an Uachtaráin: 'I cry more easily now.' She puts this down to 'the sheer range of things I have seen as High Commissioner for Human Rights', a position she held after leaving the Áras.

According to the female ministers, attitudes to politicians showing emotion have evolved. 'Well, you can imagine', says Katherine Zappone, 'what I might think of that, having been somebody who has been emotional and who has cried in public.' Zappone showed her emotions in television interviews shortly after the death of her wife, Ann Louise Gilligan, in 2017. They had spent 36 years together. In political life, Zappone believes a greater demonstration of emotional intelligence, by men as well as women, will lead to 'better policies and laws'.

Síle de Valera believes 'it's nearly a feather in men's caps politically now when they are seen to be emotional'. This, she feels, is a significant difference between her time in the Dáil, which spanned 1977 and 2007, and nowadays: 'For most of my political career you had to be very careful in even how you delivered a speech, in that you weren't seen to be too emotional. Because emotional wasn't the word that would be used by your opponents – it would be hysterical, in terms of a woman. And these terms were widely used against women. You were seen not as a strong woman, but as a hysterical woman. That's obviously changed a great deal now, I'm glad to say. Men are much more likely to show their emotions than they were. Those changes are certainly welcome, in that you can be more human.'

3

CABINET – JOINING AN EXCLUSIVE CLUB

You're getting the worst, the crankiest and the toughest of all.

GERRY COLLINS

Oh Jesus, Mary and Joseph … who?

MÁIRE GEOGHEGAN-QUINN

After the 1977 general election, Gerry Collins, a veteran Fianna Fáil politician from Limerick West, teased his party colleague Máire Geoghegan-Quinn about which department she would be assigned to and who would be her senior minister. Geoghegan-Quinn had just been appointed a junior minister (then known as a parliamentary secretary) by Taoiseach Jack Lynch. Her promotion came just two years after she was first elected a Fianna Fáil TD in Galway West in a by-election caused by the death of her father, Johnny Geoghegan. The newly-promoted TD soon found out that Desmond O'Malley was her senior minister in the Department of Industry and Commerce.

Geoghegan-Quinn says she knew little personally about O'Malley, who had been appointed Minister for Justice during the Arms Crisis almost a decade earlier and was a close associate of Lynch. The new junior minister went to meet O'Malley at his department offices: 'He introduced the secretary general and all the assistant secretaries. And he said, "Now, just to confirm that Mrs Geoghegan-Quinn is going to be responsible for the commerce division. I don't want any one of you coming to me with problems or issues or proposals. You go to her. She's effectively your minister."' It was not what she had expected, given what she had been told about O'Malley's abrasive personality. So much so that Geoghegan-Quinn says she was literally 'falling off the chair'. Later, when Ray Burke joined as a second junior minister in the department, O'Malley again set the tone: 'As far as he was concerned, there was no difference between any of us, whether we were a woman or a man didn't matter, we were the minister.'

When Lynch resigned as Fianna Fáil leader in late 1979, Geoghegan-Quinn, like O'Malley and most of her ministerial colleagues, backed George Colley over Charles Haughey. After Haughey emerged victorious, Geoghegan-Quinn was preparing for a return to the backbenches. The new Fianna Fáil leader, and Taoiseach, asked to see Geoghegan-Quinn. She predicted to her husband that, 'I will be free of everything because I'm not going to be re-appointed.' John Quinn, however, posed a hypothetical question to his wife: 'Suppose the impossible happens and he [Haughey] says to you, "Well now, Máire, I want to appoint you to cabinet. What are you going to say?"' Geoghegan-Quinn was dismissive of the proposition: 'How could I be in the cabinet? I have two young kids, I said. I'm married. I live a long way from Dublin.'

In 1979, family responsibilities would have been a serious consideration and a barrier for a woman and particularly a mother thinking about attaining senior office. Domestic arrangements would not have been such an issue for most male politicians. Today, the extent of this imbalance has narrowed but given the workload and time required of a senior politician, the impact on family life remains an issue.

As Geoghegan-Quinn arrived outside Haughey's office in Leinster House, other members of Lynch's outgoing ministerial team were already coming and going. As she waited her turn to meet the new leader, Geoghegan-Quinn remarked, 'Yeah, I'm in the right space. We are all going in to be chopped.' She was, however, proven wrong and paints a vivid picture of her interaction with Haughey: 'I walked into the office, and Charlie was sitting [with his] chair way back, arms folded, feet up on the table. And on the table was the most beautiful pristine silver tea service. He was having his tea in a beautiful china cup. And he looked at me and said, "Well, Máire, I think you and I are going to make history."' Geoghegan-Quinn was unsure what Haughey was saying: 'I looked at him and I said, "What do you mean, Taoiseach?" And he said, "I'm appointing you Minister for the Gaeltacht."' She recalls her response on receiving this dramatic news: 'Do you think, I'm able for it?' To this day, she says, 'I regret that I said that. I really do.'

Geoghegan-Quinn's response to the offer of ministerial office can perhaps be seen as an example of the insecurities many women have about their capabilities. Almost forty years later, she explains her initial doubts: 'I suppose something in my psyche at the time – or something, I think, inbred in all women at the time – was, because we had to work twice as hard as a man does, before you get credit, and even then, you don't get all the credit you deserve. It was sort of like I felt there were men more deserving of this than I was.' On hearing her response, Haughey swung his feet down from his desk and replied: 'I wouldn't have offered it to you, if I didn't know you were good enough.' As she left Haughey's office, the soon-to-be appointed Minister for the Gaeltacht was still distracted, so much so that many of her colleagues were given the wrong impression of what had happened: 'I had a big long face and everybody assumed by my demeanour that I was gone.'

Geoghegan-Quinn's appointment was historic: she was the first Irish woman since Independence in 1922 to sit at cabinet and the second since Countess Constance Markievicz attained ministerial office in 1919. Remarkably, sixty years passed between Markievicz's appointment and that of Geoghegan-Quinn. But the Galway politician's appointment was not repeated in subsequent governments headed by Haughey. He appointed her a junior minister on three different occasions (1982, 1987–9, 1989–91) but Geoghegan-Quinn had to wait until Albert Reynolds replaced Haughey as Taoiseach in 1992 before returning to the cabinet table, first as Minister for Tourism, Transport and Communications and later as Minister for Justice. The appointment to the Department of Justice was historic as Geoghegan-Quinn was the first woman to hold that ministry. She admits to having been daunted when offered the position: 'I said this is a challenge and not just for myself, but for any other woman who might aspire to be a minister in one of the non-caring ministries, I have to do a good job.' She says she enjoyed the challenge but says 'it was difficult'.

Another woman, Nora Owen, succeeded Geoghegan-Quinn in the Department of Justice. The Fine Gael politician was first elected to the Dáil in 1981, but she had to wait until the three-party Rainbow Coalition of Fine Gael, Labour and Democratic Left took office in late 1994 before being appointed a senior minister. John Bruton, a close political ally, offered her the cabinet position: 'He is quite a traditional man and he could have said, "We will give Justice, you know, with the big bad police and all that – we will give it to a man." But he didn't [...] Máire Geoghegan-Quinn had been there, and she's a pretty tough cookie. And I think, maybe John might have looked at [Geoghegan-Quinn] and said, "Well, you know, a woman can do it."' Owen says she arrived into a department now accustomed to dealing with a female minister: 'I must say I didn't find any misogyny among the officials I dealt with. They were all very respectful and made sure that I knew what was going on.' Some officials were, however, relieved for practical reasons that they were getting a second successive female minister: 'It was funny when I went into the department, they were quite pleased because they had spent a lot of time changing all the documents to "she" instead of "he". And they were pleased that they didn't have to start again.' An unforeseen consequence but for some officials, a fortuitous one.

Large-scale amendments to documents amending 'he' to 'she' could not be avoided when Geoghegan-Quinn was appointed the first female cabinet minister in over half a century in 1979. Geoghegan-Quinn admits she was 'conscious' of being the sole female among fourteen male colleagues. She recognised, however, that putting herself forward as a 'woman minister' would cause a certain amount of resentment: 'I decided I was going to be a minister first and a woman second. I was a minister who just happened to be a woman. And I was going to fight my corner. And I wasn't going to look for any favours from anybody or I wasn't going to cry or get upset if something went against me.' Nonetheless, some practical issues arose. Geoghegan-Quinn's second child, Cormac, had been born the previous July, when she was still a junior minister. After some time off work, Des O'Malley, her senior department colleague, contacted her: 'Des was on the phone. He said, "Hello," and I said, "Hello, minister." And he said, "Are you ever coming back to work?" I said, "I am, but I have a slight little problem." And he said, "What's that problem?"'

Geoghegan-Quinn was still breastfeeding. She explained that it was her intention to continue to breastfeed her baby until the end of the year, but there were no facilities in the department offices. O'Malley supported his colleague bringing the baby into the office. He said he would immediately call George Colley, who was the Minister for Finance, to see what arrangements were necessary. It seems extraordinary that the intervention of the Minister for Finance was required to organise practical arrangements for a mother returning to work, but it is one example of how in that era the political system was unprepared for mothers holding ministerial office. Within an hour of O'Malley's phone call, Colley contacted Geoghegan-Quinn.

Geoghegan-Quinn recalls that the Minister for Finance said whatever she decided 'would have be done correctly and properly' as it would then become 'the template' for other breastfeeding ministers in the future. The arrangements involved allowing a family friend, who was a student in Dublin, to mind the baby in a room next to her ministerial office: 'She did all her study and she looked after the baby. And if the baby was awake, she played with him and all the rest of it. And when the baby needed to be fed, I was sent for and I came and I fed the baby.' These arrangements continued when Geoghegan-Quinn was appointed a full cabinet member. Planning was the key: 'If I felt that there was going to be a [Dáil] vote during a cabinet meeting, which would lengthen the meeting, I would always express milk and leave a bottle of the expressed milk with the childminder. And she would give it to him in the office.'

Geoghegan-Quinn recalls the challenge of being a mother and a minister, 'packing up nappies and all that kind of stuff'. Her ministerial workload involved travelling around the country and juggling different responsibilities: 'Sometimes you might be on your way back to Galway or you might be going to Cork or to Meath or whatever. And you would always have to ring in advance, and you would get a room, a little room [to nurse the baby].' From a distance of four decades, Ireland's first cabinet minister since Independence admits: 'When I look back now I say to myself, "How in the name of God did I do that?" But it just shows you, you know, women – we are very strong characters. We don't believe we are, but we are.' While Geoghegan-Quinn initially expressed doubts when offered a cabinet position, in office she proved determined in fulfilling her duties.

❧ ❧ ❧

When the Fianna Fáil–Labour coalition was formed in 1993, Máire Geoghegan-Quinn was a member of the first ever cabinet in which two of the fifteen members were women – Niamh Bhreathnach of Labour had been appointed Minister for Education in the same government. It became a topic of conversation – not all positive – in some quarters, Geoghegan-Quinn recollects: 'I remember when the announcement was made that there were going to be two women in the cabinet, I remember all the kind of remarks being made. "Oh, two women. Sure, they will fight like cats." That was the view held in Leinster House. "Sure, they will fight like cats, two women."' Geoghegan-Quinn remembers one day overhearing two colleagues making such remarks: '[They] realised the minute they were saying it, before they even had finished the sentence – "by Jesus she's going to take our heads off".'

Bhreathnach was elected in the Spring Tide general election in November 1992 and was appointed as a member of cabinet shortly afterwards. She remembers travelling from Connemara early in the New Year when she first heard a journalist on the radio saying she was being tipped for a ministerial position. Bhreathnach found it 'gobsmacking' to be even mentioned and, in shock at the radio report, 'nearly drove the car into the bog'. As a first-time TD, Bhreathnach's ambitions were more modest – to secure a car parking space and an office: 'When I was elected, I expected to go in and sit in the backbenches.' She believes it was an advantage being a woman in the run-up to the cabinet selection – 'being a woman was part of the plus for me' – especially as Dick Spring, the Labour leader, wanted a policy programme that promoted women's issues. She says Spring's view was, '"We can't talk about women if we don't do something." He was very aware, putting a team together, that it had to include women.'

Bhreathnach sat at cabinet with Geoghegan-Quinn but says the fact that there were two female ministers in the Fianna Fáil–Labour government is where the solidarity ends. Party allegiances trumped female collegiality: 'I wouldn't say a camaraderie built up because Máire Geoghegan-Quinn was very much [in] a different party. She was very much part of the Albert Reynolds establishment.' Bhreathnach recalls sitting 'between Brian Cowen, who was very amusing, and Joe Walsh, who was very helpful. And I didn't see Máire Geoghegan-Quinn. She was up the table on the other side.' She recalls feeling the equivalent of 'the runt of the litter' at those cabinet meetings. Not only was she, as a first-time TD, the most junior politician around the table, but based on a seniority formula her seat was 'nearest the exit door'. But she was a member of the cabinet, a point she had to be quietly mindful of and reinforce when socialising with her cabinet colleagues: 'If I didn't watch it, I would end up with the wives because I was a woman. [But] my role wasn't to mind the spouses of other ministers. I had a responsibility to represent the Department of Education as a cabinet minister.'

❧ ❧ ❧

Gemma Hussey was the first woman to be appointed Minister for Education. Like Niamh Bhreathnach, the Fine Gael politician's rise to ministerial office came early in her Dáil career. Hussey says she was 'astonished' when Garret FitzGerald promoted her to cabinet in December 1982. Other politicians were also taken aback that Hussey, who had won a Dáil seat the previous February – in the first of two elections in 1982 – had been elevated so rapidly. In his memoir, former Labour minister Barry Desmond says one of Hussey's predecessors in the Department of Education, her party colleague John Boland, was personally of the view that she had 'hand-bagged' him out of the ministerial position.[27] Hussey has little time for this observation, which she views as sexist. Describing the remark as 'extraordinary', she says John Boland 'was a tough cookie. And for anybody to handbag him would have been impossible.'

As a member of the second Garret FitzGerald-led Fine Gael–Labour coalition in the 1980s, Hussey was in office during a challenging economic and political era. She felt under additional pressure as the only woman around the cabinet table. She admits to being 'so conscious of the fact that I was going to be judged not only as a woman, as a feminist. I was aware that out in the country there were all these women and that if I made a mess of things, people would say, "Ah, well, sure she's a woman and what can you expect?" Now it mightn't happen nowadays, but it would have happened in those days. And I didn't want to let women down. So I had that extra pressure on me.'

Hussey's appointment as a minister, coming shortly after Máire Geoghegan-Quinn's breakthrough promotion in 1979 – and Eileen Desmond in 1981 – provoked what she describes as a 'culture shock' among several male ministerial colleagues. Hussey believes that aside from the new experience of having a female minister at cabinet, some of her male colleagues had never previously had a serious political discussion with a female counterpart, largely due to the wider absence of women in political life. At one cabinet meeting when reducing the cost of food subsidies was under discussion, Jim Mitchell, the late Fine Gael minister, was calculating the impact on the price of rashers and sausages. He turned directly to his female ministerial colleague asking, 'Gemma, come here, what is the price of a pound of rashers?' Hussey, who describes Mitchell as 'an awfully nice man' but traditional in his outlook, did not have time to even offer an answer. Garret FitzGerald interjected: 'How would that woman know any more about a price for a pound of rashers than you would? She is out working all of the hours that God gives, like you are. So why would she know anything about the price of a pound of rashers?' Hussey recalls there was laughter around the cabinet table as the Taoiseach's remarks 'more or less told Jim [and] put him in his box'. She views FitzGerald as a feminist in how he backed her at cabinet when she was a minister.

At some of the initial meetings of the coalition cabinet, the new Minister for Education also found that she had to be assertive so as to ensure she did not end up 'getting stuck' making tea for some of her male ministerial colleagues – a small but symbolic act. She recalls a conversation with Peter Barry, who was Minister for Foreign Affairs in the 1982–87 government and a well-known businessman from Cork whose family owned Barry's Tea: 'I think Peter thought I was going to make the tea. He was a sweet man but he was very traditional. And he never liked me. I remember saying [as] a joke to Peter, "Listen, you're the one that makes the great tea."'

A decade after Hussey left government in 1987, another woman who held senior ministerial office was equally conscious that the tea-making duties were not delegated to the female members of cabinet. Fianna Fáil's Síle de Valera says she was never asked but she may have partly contributed to that outcome: 'If there was a male colleague that made the tea and handed me a cup, I would have said, thank you very much. But I wasn't because it was associated with so-called "women's work". I would make the point by not putting on the kettle as it were.' Among the female ministers, there are different views on the matter – another former Fianna Fáil minister, Mary Hanafin, says her approach was very straightforward: 'If you were the first in, I was happy, "Here, do you want a cup of tea or whatever."' As she explains, 'I wanted to be busy, you know.' But she is equally keen to stress that 'I'm not saying I made the tea all the time. I didn't. But I had no problem making the tea.'

❖ ❖ ❖

No female politician has served as long or for as continuous a term at cabinet as Mary Harney. In total, the former Progressive Democrats leader spent fourteen years at cabinet between 1997 and 2011. She also has the distinction of being the first woman to be appointed Tánaiste. Harney's ministerial career could have been even longer had she not been overlooked for a cabinet appointment when the first Fianna Fáil–Progressive Democrats coalition was formed in 1989. Following a deal between the Fianna Fáil leader Charles Haughey and Des O'Malley, his Progressive Democrats counterpart, the smaller coalition party secured two cabinet seats and one junior ministerial position. O'Malley and Bobby Molloy, a Progressive Democrats TD from Galway West, filled the two cabinet posts. Harney was given the junior job. 'I was a little taken aback that I wasn't a [cabinet] minister then,' she admits decades later. 'Bobby had the experience, maybe age. I don't know. I have never discussed that with Des. But I was a little disappointed, because we had started the party together.' She puts the decision down to political considerations: 'It's not always necessarily the best people that always get the positions. Geography and gender now seem to play as big a part as ability.

And I think that's a pity.' Geography and loyalty however, have outweighed gender, which is clearly demonstrated by the number of women ministers, even in recent times.

As a junior minister in the Department of the Environment from 1989 to 1992, Harney had responsibility for environmental protection. Relations with Pádraig Flynn, her senior ministerial colleague, in the department were not good, to say the least. In his memoir, Des O'Malley says Flynn 'treated [Harney] like absolute dirt'.[28] Harney recalls that 'a special door' was opened in the Custom House where the Department of the Environment was based. This meant she came and went via a side door, not the front entrance. Her offices were also located away from the where the main business of the department took place. The symbolism of this is not lost on Harney: 'Now that wasn't a big issue for me, but it was a symbol of you know, keep her far away from the centre of action.' She believes the Fianna Fáil politician's attitude was motivated more by his hostility to the coalition arrangement than to her being a woman. But Harney also says the Mayo TD had 'gender issues'. These attitudes were evident in how he would speak to her: 'He would talk to you as if you were one of his children,' she says, recalling remarks such as, 'You are like my daughter. What's wrong with you?' Flynn, she says, was not an easy person to work with, for a woman: 'Ironically, one of his advisors was a woman. But I think when it came to a woman politician he didn't really feel that was your place.'

Harney succeeded O'Malley as Progressive Democrats leader in 1993 and led the party into a coalition arrangement with Fianna Fáil after the 1997 general election. Bertie Ahern became Taoiseach and Harney was appointed Tánaiste and Minister for Enterprise, Trade and Employment. Securing an economic ministry was important to her. 'That's the one I wanted. The Tánaiste was a bonus,' she recalls. She was conscious, though, of the significance of being the first woman to hold the position of Tánaiste: 'There was a bit made of that. I have to be honest, for the first three or four months, when I was at an event and somebody said, "The Tánaiste", I would immediately think of [the previous Tánaiste, Labour's] Dick Spring. The Tánaiste was so associated with him, that I used to forget it was me.' The role gave Harney additional political clout beyond being Progressive Democrats leader and the holder of a senior economic ministerial position: 'It got a lot of coverage, and obviously it has a significance in government. You deputise for the Taoiseach, so there's the public side of the Dáil and Leaders' Questions. But then there was the private side, meeting international delegations and being included in a lot of stuff by virtue of being Tánaiste.'

Most of Harney's time at cabinet was during Ahern's tenure as Taoiseach (1997–2008). They formed a good working relationship: 'It didn't matter whether you were a woman or a man. He got on with it [and was] very pragmatic.' Mary O'Rourke has a similar view of the politician who appointed her deputy leader of Fianna Fáil in 1994. She was the first woman to hold that position in the party: 'Bertie was full of equality. He didn't realise it, but he was … we had a very, very good relationship.'

O'Rourke was first appointed to cabinet by Haughey in 1987 as Minister for Education. She found Haughey paternalistic at times in his approach. During her tenure in the Department of Education, O'Rourke did not mind being the only female minister at the cabinet table, although on occasion she had to deal with boyish behaviour. The minority Fianna Fáil government oversaw a policy of severe austerity politics, labelled 'fiscal rectitude', and all departments budgets were significantly reduced. Education was no different, but O'Rourke wanted to develop educational resources, including appointing teachers to liaise with the parents of children who were struggling in the classroom or having trouble with attendance. She prepared a memo for cabinet and circulated it to her ministerial colleagues. Haughey asked her to outline the proposal at a subsequent cabinet meeting. Ray MacSharry, the Minister for Finance, with whom she 'would become great friends with afterwards', was not impressed: 'Up pipes MacSharry, saying, "Taoiseach, these are teachers that don't teach."' Another Fianna Fáil minister started to snigger at what he thought was O'Rourke's naivety. 'They were like boys in a schoolyard,' she says. Looking back, she believes some of her male colleagues thought she would 'get her comeuppance. Imagine bringing that to cabinet when it's cut, cut, cut'. But Haughey allowed O'Rourke to proceed to make her case and the cabinet eventually approved a number of pilot schemes.

O'Rourke also remembers some of her male colleagues using very colourful language. 'They would "fuck" and they would "feck" and they would "fuck" and they would "feck" and they would "shite" – which is a word I hate – across the table.' She recalls that Albert 'was a great curser', while Ray MacSharry used expletives 'on and off'. When Haughey cursed in front of her, he would say, "Excuse me, Mary, we shouldn't be at that kind of talk in front of you."' O'Rourke had her reply: 'Do you think I came from a nunnery?' 'Oh sure, I suppose, Mary,' Haughey said.

In 1997, O'Rourke was one of three women who sat at the cabinet table – Harney had just been appointed along with another ministerial newcomer, Síle de Valera. Having served on the Fianna Fáil front bench from 1994 to 1997, de Valera was 'very emotional' at being asked by Ahern to become Minister for Arts, Heritage, Gaeltacht and the Islands. She did not notice 'cliques' within the cabinet but recalls that Harney was an ally in the sense that she was 'always supportive of you as a woman. It wasn't anything overt. But you knew that support was there. In that she would listen very intently to what you would have to say or if you brought a delegation into her.'

While Ahern promoted de Valera to cabinet in 1997, she was dropped as a senior minister when he appointed his second ministerial team after the 2002 general election: 'I was very disappointed, because I had spent five years in opposition and five years in government [as Minister for] the Arts, Heritage [Gaeltacht and the Islands]. And I would have loved to have continued. But it wasn't to be. In fairness to Bertie Ahern, he said I could have any minister of state position I wished. And he smiled, I remember [him] saying, "I think it might be education, would it, Síle?" And I said, "Yes. I would love that."'

Around this time, another female Fianna Fáil politician was taken aside by a colleague and advised to kick-start a ministerial career by having a chat with Ahern. Mary Coughlan had been a TD since 1987 and, having been overlooked for ministerial office after the Fianna Fáil–Progressive Democrats coalition was formed in 1997, felt she had served a long apprenticeship in Leinster House. Around 2000, a party colleague advised her to be proactive: 'Mary, it's about time you got up the ladder. You have served a long time in the House. You are not going to do it if you stand back and let it go past you.' Spurred on, Coughlan arranged an appointment with Ahern to press her case: 'I said, "Look, I know there's loads of people. I'm not putting you under pressure, but I don't want it ever to be said that I'm not interested." He said, "That's fair enough." And I went on my merry way to do whatever I had to do and then shortly afterwards I got a phone call.' Her colleague's advice proved useful on this occasion: Coughlan was appointed a junior minister in February 2001. Sixteen months later, she was in cabinet. She served as Minister for Social and Family Affairs from 2002 to 2004 before moving to the Department of Agriculture and Food (2004–08). She served as Tánaiste from 2008 to 2011, and in those years was also Minister for Enterprise, Trade and Employment (2008–10) and subsequently Education (2010–11). She was even Minister for Health and Children for six weeks in early 2011 having been assigned the additional ministerial portfolio by Brian Cowen in the dying days of the government that collapsed at the height of the economic crisis.

Given her constituency work in Donegal, Coughlan was very familiar with the activities of the Department of Social and Family Affairs. But she was not long in her new ministerial role when she was confronted with the need to reduce the departmental budget by €50 million. Some of her cabinet colleagues were very supportive: 'Mary Harney was very good to me, and Cowen and other people were very good at trying to find a way of easing [the pressure]. The view was you do one big hit and take some scheme out of it altogether, or you try and do a little bit to lessen the blow on a number of schemes.' She chose the latter option but faced severe criticism from groups representing widows and widowers, aggrieved that their entitlements were being cut. 'I got slaughtered,' Coughlan says bluntly. 'I think I was known as the "wicked witch of the north-west". All those photographs of me on a broom.' There was also 'a vicious altercation' when an opposition politician approached her in the restaurant in Leinster House saying, '"I thought you were a person who would empathise with these things. Your mother is a widow," and all this craic.' Coughlan felt like responding, 'Would you ever just get off the soapbox?' She believes a male minister might have received similar treatment, but 'not as bad'.

Coughlan's switch to the Department of Agriculture during Ahern's ministerial reshuffle in 2004 came as a real surprise to her: 'They were nerve-racking days. Sitting, waiting on a phone call, it's not good for the health. But anyway, he brought me in and he said, "I'm taking a big risk on this one." And I thought,

"Oh God, what is he going to do to me now?" He says, "I'm going to appoint you to Agriculture, and you are going to be the first ever woman Minister for Agriculture. Because I think you are well fit to do it. And it's about time there was a woman in the department." Coughlan replied, "'Thanks very much, and I hope I don't let you down." I was hoping to get out of that room as quick as I could, to get my breath.'

Coming from a rural constituency, Coughlan had an interest in agricultural policy and knew many industry leaders. But she recognised she was taking over as the political figurehead of a 'hugely male-orientated industry'. There were some doubts about 'a woman representing the hills and dales of Donegal' being responsible for the sector. She remembers getting off to 'a very bad start' when one man 'turned around to me and he says, "What would a bloody woman from the north-west know about my problems?"' Coughlan worked hard to convert those who had doubts. She hosted meetings with industry figures and travelled to functions and events all over the country: 'You would get the fella with the one tooth and the big kiss and about six inches of cow dung on their wellingtons. But sure, look, they were good people.'

Like many women who have held cabinet positions, Coughlan was conscious of walking into a room where she was the only woman but, she says, 'I work very well with men and I get on very well with men. So I enjoyed the challenge of working with people.' While Coughlan's ministerial career spans nine years and five different departments, it was her appointment as Tánaiste and Minister for Enterprise, Trade and Employment in 2008 that received most attention and criticism. She says up to that point, she would have been 'a fairly popular person, within the parliamentary party'. However, following her elevation by Brian Cowen when he appointed his ministerial team after succeeding Ahern in 2008, there were colleagues 'who would have cut my throat'. She thinks that any of her male colleagues who found themselves in such a position would have been treated similarly, as this was about promotional prospects and party hierarchy, not gender, although it may have been an aggravating factor.

Having been comfortable in the Departments of Social Affairs and later Agriculture, Coughlan was now under huge pressure and considerable scrutiny in her new economic brief: 'The world economy didn't suit me. People had to do a 360 in a lot of departments that they weren't accustomed to. And the first thing is, we had to take so much money out of the economy. For anybody at political level, and within a department, to do that is just the most difficult thing you could ever do. Everybody likes to protect their own patch, either their own department or their own section within the department. And that was very difficult.'

❧ ❧ ❧

While the appointment of a new cabinet is an historic and significant event, it's also very personal for those promoted, demoted or overlooked. On the day of the announcement, TDs with aspirations of political elevation are on high alert and literally watching for any sign that a promotion is coming their way. For incumbent ministers, there is the anxiety of holding onto their position around the cabinet table. On this day of ritual and drama, Leinster House is a flurry of activity with politicians and the media seeking out any information on what decisions are being taken by the Taoiseach of the day.

In the aftermath of the collapse of Albert Reynolds's Fianna Fáil–Labour coalition in late 1994, the new government was formed without a general election taking place for the first time in Irish history. John Bruton led Fine Gael into office in a coalition arrangement with Labour and Democratic Left. Frances Fitzgerald was a new Fine Gael TD ensconced in the Dáil office of veteran party colleague Jim Mitchell. From their office window, they could see every movement on the glass bridge that joins Leinster House with Government Buildings. It was a perfect vantage point from which to see cabinet formation in practice. Mitchell offered a running commentary on the political careers being made and broken: 'The civil servants were really scurrying around, looking for people and to bring them over. And Jim was there saying, "Oh no. Gay isn't being called, I'm not being called."'

After a decade as a TD, Fitzgerald lost her seat in the 2002 general election. She was an unsuccessful candidate again in 2007 but having spent the following four years in the Seanad, she returned to the Dáil in 2011 and was appointed to cabinet. Over the following six years she held three different ministries (Children and Youth Affairs, 2011–14), Justice and Equality (2014–17) and Business, Enterprise and Innovation (2017). When Enda Kenny was forming the Fine Gael–Labour government in 2011, Fitzgerald 'hadn't a clue' which ministry she might get nor that a new Department of Children and Youth Affairs was going to be established. Following the resignation of Alan Shatter as Minister for Justice in May 2014, Kenny contacted her: 'I got a phone call the night before saying, "I will call you early in the morning," without telling me [which department she was being assigned to] and then [Kenny] rang me very early in the morning and said, "Can you meet me at 9 a.m.?" When the Fine Gael–Independent minority coalition took office in May 2016, Fitzgerald became the first female Fine Gael politician to be appointed Tánaiste, a position she retained when Leo Varadkar succeeded Kenny as Taoiseach just over a year later. She resigned from cabinet in November 2017 in the midst of a controversy involving her department and the handling of a garda whistle-blower. By that stage, she had become the longest-serving female Fine Gael minister.

Fitzgerald firmly holds the view that the number of senior female ministers at cabinet 'makes a difference'. She was one of two women – the other, Labour's Joan Burton – appointed to cabinet in 2011. Attorney General Máire Whelan also sat at the cabinet table. For Fitzgerald, having Burton there was important: 'I was always pleased that Joan was there, for example. A different party, but we had lots of things that we would support one another in.' Burton agrees: 'When you get into the cabinet, you have to put your hand up and you have to say, "I have something to say." Otherwise, if you were just going to be the equivalent of a doormat, people will happily let you lie there at the edge of the door and say nothing.' Burton says she was determined 'that my voice carried the same weight, and more weight. So I was always a contributor to the cabinet. Now that may have been a pain in the arse to other people.'

Fitzgerald has found that female ministers had to be not only assertive at the cabinet table but 'overassertive' to make their case on issues under consideration: 'I have had the experience again and again and again in cabinet and elsewhere, of putting forward an idea, of having a man put forward the same idea some time later and the reference being made back to the man, not to me.' The former Tánaiste says 'out of amusement' she decided to highlight this trend to some of her ministerial colleagues: 'I would say, "Are you monitoring it?" and they would laugh. And they wouldn't have seen it. They wouldn't have noticed it. It happens all the time. And it happens in cabinet.'

❧ ❧ ❧

Following a cabinet reshuffle in 2014, two more women were appointed as senior ministers – Heather Humphreys (Fine Gael) and Jan O'Sullivan (Labour). At four out of the fifteen positions at cabinet, this is the highest number of female ministers to date. With more women around the table, Frances Fitzgerald observed new dynamics in the room: 'It certainly makes it easier for women to contribute and to be taken seriously,' she says. Humphreys says she was not conscious of the male dominance around the table, but her previous professional experiences have shown that the dynamics change when more women are involved: 'I have worked in banking, in the credit union movement. And there's always been a predominance of men at board tables, always more men than women. So this didn't come as any big surprise to me.' But, she says: 'I think women are more conciliatory. That can help, it can help defuse meetings sometimes, if you are more conciliatory and you try to bring people with you.'

In her senior and junior ministerial roles, Mary Mitchell O'Connor of Fine Gael has been struck by the absence of women: 'I have gone into rooms, and I ask, "Are there any women?" [In] nearly every meeting that I go to there's a majority of men in the room.' However, she says she did not think about the number of female ministers around the cabinet table when she was appointed a senior minister in 2016: 'We were conscious of getting a job done. There was serious business and that's the way of work at the cabinet table. It wasn't that I was sitting at the cabinet table, thinking, "Oh, I'm a woman, and there's three other women." You know, my job was to deliver jobs and employment. And that's what I did.' In a similar vein, Independent TD Katherine Zappone, who was also appointed to cabinet in 2016, says she is more conscious of her political status than being a female minister: 'I'm very conscious of the fact that I'm a woman. But does it make a difference? I think it's the non-aligned Independent that makes more of a difference or that one can see explicitly.'

Fine Gael's Regina Doherty sees no distinction between her male and female ministerial colleagues. She was appointed Government Chief Whip in 2016 before becoming Minister for Employment Affairs and Social Protection in 2017. She says, 'Now do I look around the table and see a few women and a load of men? I actually don't. I just look around the table and see different views, different opinions. We all have allies in different places. And it depends on the topic – you might be my ally today if we are talking about apples, but if we are talking about oranges next Tuesday it mightn't be you.'

Beyond the cabinet room, Máire Geoghegan-Quinn says she was very self-conscious at official events at the absence of women in attendance especially when she was Minister for Justice: 'All the key people in the key positions in the organisation were all men. I don't think a male minister would even notice that there were so few women around. He wouldn't be interested in that, or it wouldn't sort of dawn on him.' When Mary Harney first arrived at the Department of Enterprise, Trade and Employment in 1997, she was struck at the 'exclusively male management team': 'Even the senior people in the IDA, Enterprise Ireland, the people I engaged with went on trade missions, went on IDA promotional trips [were] all men.' She recalls that from her nomination to the Seanad in 1977 she 'was in a very male environment all the time during my political career'. But this gender profile changed when she became Minister for Health and Children in 2004: 'Health was the reverse. There were a lot more women at a senior level there [...] So it was a completely different experience, from a gender perspective. Did I see any difference in the approach, between men and women? Probably not.'

For Mary Hanafin, gender came into play when one senior official asked whether to call her 'Minister, Mary or Ms …' Astonished at the question, Hanafin replied, 'You can call me whatever you like, but you are not calling me Ms.' Hanafin remembers her elevation to a senior ministerial position in 2004. It was particularly poignant as her husband Eamon Leahy had died the previous year. The Dún Laoghaire politician had been a junior minister from 2000 to 2002, after which she was appointed Government Chief Whip. In 2004, Bertie Ahern called Hanafin into his office and asked, 'Do you think you are able for this?' She replied, 'Of course I am. I'm a strong person. I'm great now and I'm a big girl.' As she attempted to reassure Ahern she was ready for a full cabinet position, he confirmed he was appointing her Minister for Education. 'I burst into tears,' she recalls, adding that Ahern was 'kindness personified'. Later, in the Dáil chamber as the Taoiseach was confirming his new ministerial appointment, Hanafin recalls seeing 92 messages on her phone: 'Of course, so many of them were from Eamon's colleagues and friends, and that meant a huge amount to me.' It was also a big day for Hanafin's father Des, who first won a seat in the Seanad in 1969 and had departed national politics in 2002. Having tried unsuccessfully to win a Dáil seat in Tipperary North in 1977 and 1981, ministerial office was never a possibility for him. With the elevation of his daughter, one relation said, 'That's the day that Des thinks he was appointed a minister.'

At cabinet, Hanafin was one of three women around the table but does not believe there was a particular camaraderie: 'I don't think there was collegiality between the women. But, you see, the cabinet broke down, not on male–female, but on Fianna Fáil–Progressive Democrats party [affiliation].' It is hardly surprising that party allegiance was the important binding factor, a view shared by other female ministers. Jan O'Sullivan says she was closest to her own party colleagues in the 2011–16 Fine Gael–Labour coalition, although female ministers were generally 'pretty supportive of each other … [especially] on particular issues that we felt strongly about'. Although it has been shown time and time again that any potential sisterhood rarely breaches party lines.

❧ ❧ ❧

No woman has yet served as Minister for Foreign Affairs or Minister for Finance, generally seen as two of the most powerful and influential cabinet briefs beyond the position of Taoiseach. Joan Burton probably came closest to being the first woman to serve as a senior minister in the Department of Finance. Burton was first elected to the Dáil in 1992 and was a junior minister from 1992 to 1997. She lost her seat in 1997 but regained it five years later, becoming a senior member of Labour's front bench and was the party's finance spokesperson from 2002 to 2011. She secured the role after Pat Rabbitte succeeded Ruairi Quinn at the top of the party in 2002: 'I sat down with Pat Rabbitte after he became leader and he said, – being Pat, who is very amusing – "I suppose, I have to ask you what would you like to do?" And I said to him, "There's only one thing I can do, and I should do, and that's be finance spokesperson." Now I think he was a bit taken aback, because I'm not sure if he had expected me to say that quite so bluntly. But in for a penny in for a pound. So I left the room finance spokesperson of the Labour Party.'

From the opposition benches, Burton first shadowed Fianna Fáil's Charlie McCreevy and later Brian Cowen and Brian Lenihan as the Irish economy moved from boom to bust between 2002 and 2011. In the aftermath of strong electoral gains for both Fine Gael and Labour in 2011, Burton knew a cabinet position was probable when Enda Kenny and Eamon Gilmore agreed to lead their respective parties into government. But unlike her previous conversation with Pat Rabbitte, she left the room following a discussion with Gilmore, 'extremely disappointed'. Burton says their conversation came late on the day when cabinet positions were being filled: 'The longer the day went on, the less confident I felt about what I would be offered. I still thought I would be offered, at a very minimum, an economic ministry.' But heading the Department of Finance, or even the consolation of another economic ministry, was not on offer: 'I remember the conversation. It was fairly brief. I may have been close to the last appointment that was offered. And I had worked out that because it was kind of a woman's area, I was going to be offered Social Protection.' She recalls a combination of personal disappointment and being left 'stunned and appalled' that Fine Gael was dominating the main positions in cabinet: 'It was a very unbalanced coalition in which Fine Gael had Taoiseach and Minister for Finance and Minister for Jobs. I just couldn't get over it.' She gave some thought to not accepting Gilmore's offer of the Department of Social Protection but ultimately accepted while warning her party leader that it would be an 'unpopular decision'. The reaction was swift. When the new ministers walked into the Dáil for the first time and Kenny formally announced his ministerial line-up, Burton could hear her mobile phone: 'I could feel my bag vibrating. It would be called a Twitter storm [nowadays], but I was having a messaging storm on my phone.'

In July 2014, Burton succeeded Gilmore as Labour leader, the first woman to hold that position and the first female member of her party to be appointed Tánaiste. In the reshuffle that followed, she promoted her colleague Jan O'Sullivan as Minister for Education, bringing the number of female ministers at cabinet to four – the highest to date (September 2018). On securing cabinet rank, O'Sullivan says, 'Joan would be a very strong believer in women, you know, women being given powerful and responsible roles. [...] Joan is a strong personality. And she would have been quite assertive about how she thought things should be done. But having said that, she would have been supportive of me, as a woman in the role I was in. And I think of other women within the party as well.' Before she was appointed a senior minister, O'Sullivan had attended cabinet meetings as a 'super junior' minister. Burton's predecessor as Labour leader and Tánaiste, Eamon Gilmore, had appointed O'Sullivan to the post in 2011, and interestingly she believes he was 'consciously feminist' in his attitudes and 'probably the most woman-friendly' of all the party leaders she has worked with.

❧ ❧ ❧

Mary Mitchell O'Connor says she will never forget the day in 2016 she was appointed Minister for Jobs, Enterprise and Innovation by Enda Kenny: 'I suppose I was surprised. I was genuinely elated. It's a huge honour. My parents were both alive at the time. And it was a huge honour for my sons. And, especially for someone that ... I was new to politics. I was a newbie.' Despite throwing herself into the job, Mitchell O'Connor lasted only thirteen months as a senior minister. In the summer of 2017, she was demoted when Leo Varadkar succeeded Kenny as Fine Gael leader and Taoiseach. This caught many by surprise, as she had supported Varadkar in the Fine Gael leadership contest. There was a consolation prize in her appointment as a 'super junior' minister with responsibility for higher education with the right to attend cabinet. It was reported that she was originally offered another junior position but turned it down: 'I'm not commenting on what I was originally offered. If you look at the history of politics, there are good days and bad days. That probably wasn't my best day.'

Cabinet promotions and demotions can be viewed like a game of political snakes and ladders with some surprises along the way. Heather Humphreys falls into the latter category. In July 2014 Humphreys got an unexpected call to go to the Taoiseach's office. The outcome of the meeting took most in the political system, including the woman herself, by surprise. Humphreys was a first-term TD, having won a Dáil seat in Cavan–Monaghan in the 2011 general election. She had no expectation of being offered a junior position, not to mind being asked to join the cabinet.

During Kenny's ministerial reshuffle, Humphreys had speculated over coffee with several Fine Gael colleagues in Leinster House about who would be in and who would be out. She recalls the gossip and then saying, 'Lads, I'm away. I have work to do. It's not going to affect me.' Back in her Dáil office, Humphreys was making phone calls and dealing with constituency issues when she received a call on her mobile phone. The Taoiseach wanted to see her: 'What actually went through my head was talk on the radio that maybe I would be considered for a junior position. So I thought to myself, well, he's probably bringing over people that he's not giving jobs to. I thought I was going to get some kind of a pep talk. I genuinely didn't think I was going to get an appointment.' When Humphreys met Kenny, he informed her that he was appointing her Minister for Arts, Heritage and the Gaeltacht: 'I was kind of shocked. I didn't know what to say. I thanked him very much. And I said, "I would do my best. And I would try not to let him down." I remember he said to me, "Now, Heather, when you go out that door things will change. They will never be the same again."'

After leaving Government Buildings, she met her party colleague Patrick O'Donovan, who had been listening to speculation about the reshuffle on the radio. He told her the names being mentioned for promotion, including another colleague being touted as Minister for the Arts and Heritage. Humphreys replied, 'No, me.' She remembers O'Donovan replying, 'What?', to which she said, 'It's me.' O'Donovan was soon dispatched to help her prepare for the unexpected but impending official announcement of her promotion: 'I had a new jacket in the car. And I said, "Run out and get me that jacket, Patrick, please." So he ran out to the car and brought me in the stuff. I changed and then I was ready.'

While Humphreys's elevation blindsided most political pundits and politicians including herself, many suspected that her party colleague Regina Doherty felt overlooked in the 2014 reshuffle. Doherty remembers being under scrutiny at the time: 'What everybody thought was, "The cocky cow thought that she should have been promoted" [...] And that's what was reported. Sure, I was only here for three years. How would I ever have thought I was going to be promoted?' A first-time TD in 2011, Doherty is known as being outspoken. In 2014, she highlighted the absence of any Fine Gael women in the junior ministerial line-up following Kenny's mid-term government reshuffle. Doherty met Kenny a few days after her remarks were reported in the media. She describes him as 'an incredibly warm person'. The then Fine Gael leader advised her, she says, 'that I was only in the door, and that I had a bright future ahead, and not to be wanting to run before, you know, and all warm and, and lovely stuff.'

Doherty's outspoken comments did not affect her career trajectory – two years later in 2016, she got her first ministerial breakthrough when Kenny appointed her Government Chief Whip; a little over a year later, Leo Varadkar promoted her to Minister for Employment Affairs and Social Protection. But Doherty was not certain about her promotional prospects under

Varadkar, who she had supported in the Fine Gael leadership contest: 'I couldn't have been 100 per cent sure that Leo was going to include me in cabinet. I had obviously hoped that the worst thing that could happen was that he would leave me as Chief Whip.' On the eve of the cabinet appointments, Doherty was debating with her husband whether or not to ring Varadkar. Having opted not to call, the couple went to a local restaurant for dinner when her phone rang: 'It was Leo, and he said, "You are the only person that hasn't rung me."' Doherty replied, 'Well, I reckoned that you probably had enough on your plate.' She didn't tell him the full story: 'I certainly wasn't going to admit to him that I was afraid to ring him.' In a short two- to three-minute conversation, Varadkar asked Doherty for her thoughts on portfolios: 'I said, "I will do whatever you want me to do." Like, total eejit, right? And he said, "That's game ball, I will talk to you tomorrow." So he didn't give anything away. And I, like a total eejit, having been asked, would I like to be the Minister for Coffee said, no, no, sure whatever you want me to do.' Doherty says she sat at the dinner table thinking, 'I am an awful gobshite. What will I do?' She decided to text Varadkar. Her message read 'I know I said I would do anything, but if Carlsberg did reshuffles, I would love Social Protection.' 'He replied "Really? Because most people think that it's a certain type of portfolio," and he went on to tell me, "but it's really great" because obviously he was the Minister for Social Protection. And that was it.'

There was still the nerve-racking wait for the formal offer of a job. While the new Taoiseach was calling people to his office to deliver good and bad news, the Dáil was still sitting. Doherty's family had gathered in Leinster House: 'My poor mother is having a heart attack upstairs in the gallery. So she says, "I got all my knickers in a knot."' Eventually Doherty was asked to go to the Taoiseach's office: 'I kind of knew from the night before.

He wasn't going to call and then disappoint me. But things can happen during that day.' Varadkar delivered the news – he was appointing Doherty to Employment and Social Protection: 'I was cockahoo, ten foot tall, deadly.' She recalls that all her family except her father were in the Dáil gallery waiting for the new ministers to follow the Taoiseach into the chamber, as is tradition: 'My daddy was down at the coffee dock on his own, watching it on the telly, because he wasn't well and he wasn't up to the crowd that was upstairs in the gallery. And I legged it from the Taoiseach's department down to my daddy to get a hug, to tell him.'

Doherty joined three other women, including Katherine Zappone, at cabinet. The Independent TD was appointed Minister for Children and Youth Affairs by Enda Kenny when the Fine Gael–Independent minority government was formed in 2016. She was a newly elected Independent TD, having spent the previous five years in the Seanad. The Labour leader Eamon Gilmore had put her name forward as a Taoiseach's nominee as part of the 2011 Fine Gael–Labour coalition deal. Although Kenny had appointed her to the Seanad, there had been some tension when Zappone opposed the government's referendum to abolish the Seanad in 2013: 'He [Taoiseach Enda Kenny] didn't talk to me for four or five months afterwards, didn't say a goddamn word to me ... [he was] very sore about that.' Despite this friction, Zappone voted for Kenny's re-election as Taoiseach in 2016. She says she respected 'his willingness to try to get a government together. I felt his efforts were genuine.' As part of the deal, Zappone was offered a seat at the cabinet table, with several Independent TDs taking ministerial positions alongside Fine Gael politicians. Zappone did not know what portfolio she was getting until Kenny told her that she was being appointed to the Department of Children and Youth Affairs.

Zappone admits to being conscious of the number of women around the table, and believes if there were more female ministers it 'would make a difference in terms of, probably the atmosphere'. At cabinet, she says her male colleagues listen to her and take what she says seriously. But she notices that the male voices dominate and tend to get referenced more in discussions: 'It's normal for the male voice to take up most of the time [...] you know all this, that the men, when they do speak, they refer back to another man's point, when in fact you have made the point.' So, she believes 'it would be easier for me to bring my voice more regularly to the table if there were half and half [gender representation].' Nevertheless, Zappone has also seen how male voices have contributed to sensitive issues. She recalls the cabinet debate on the Eighth Amendment, the prohibition on abortion inserted into the Irish Constitution in 1983 and repealed in a referendum in May 2018: 'Many men drew on the experience of close women in their lives in terms of their reflection that impacted their decision and their position now. A lot of them. That's a change.' She believes that 'that's a success for those of us who have said for so long, "listen to the voices of women, to their experiences" and so on.'

A little over a year after Kenny asked her to join government, Zappone found herself working with a new Fine Gael Taoiseach. She says Leo Varadkar 'is a shier man than Enda', who is 'very comfortable with women'. Humphreys, who also served under both men in cabinet, says 'Leo is probably more direct and to the point.' Regina Doherty highlights age and length of service when making comparisons. Kenny had been Fine Gael leader for 'donkeys' years' before she was elected to the Dáil, not to mind appointed a minister. As a result, Doherty never felt his equal: 'Now, I'm not saying I'm Leo's equal, but I'm a hell of a lot more equal with Leo than I ever was with Enda. There was always a reverence and a respect for Enda. Before Leo was ever our leader, Leo was my friend. I would have conversations with Leo that I never would have been able to have with Enda.'

Her party colleague Frances Fitzgerald had conversations with both party leaders about the number of women at cabinet: 'I have always felt that getting to 30 per cent or 40 per cent makes a difference. I would have said that I would like to see more women.' She says both men considered gender representation to be important but that they were also balancing a variety of other demands: 'They obviously were conscious of it. But they would usually say, you know we are trying to balance x, y and z. There are always balances, there are always loyalties, there is always geography. It's very competitive.'

❖ ❖ ❖

Josepha Madigan's promotion to cabinet by Leo Varadkar in November 2017 did not result in an increase in the total number of women at cabinet. Her elevation followed the resignation of another female minister, Frances Fitzgerald, who stepped down in the midst of a political crisis caused by the fallout from a garda whistle-blower controversy that threatened to prematurely end the life of the Fine Gael-led minority coalition. Fitzgerald's departure prevented an early general election being called but left Varadkar with decisions about a cabinet reshuffle. On becoming Taoiseach five months previous, Varadkar had ruled out promoting first-time TDs to ministerial office. That had put an end to the aspirations of newly elected TDs like Madigan, who had been elected in Dublin–Rathdown in the February 2016 general election. By November 2017, the criteria for cabinet selection had changed, prompted in part by the clamour over the low number of women in ministerial ranks.

While Madigan admits to having had hopes of a junior position the prospect of a senior ministry was not on her mind: 'I had just dropped the kids to school and he [Varadkar] rang me about 8.20 in the morning. And I missed the call because I wasn't expecting a call. So then I rang him back and then he asked me.' As Varadkar spoke on the phone about cabinet appointments, Madigan says she 'nearly crashed the car'. She did not have a chance to tell her own children as they were already at school by the time the Taoiseach had contacted her. She was so unprepared for the news that she did not even know that she could bring them to the Phoenix Park to witness her receiving her seal of office from the president.

That afternoon, Madigan's mother collected her two sons from school. In the car, they listened as Madigan was interviewed on radio: 'They actually heard me on RTÉ, and I said, "I'm not even sure if my children know"'. Madigan says her mother cried when she first heard the news. She had recently suffered the bereavements of her husband, Paddy, and youngest daughter, Edwina. Madigan's own thoughts also turned to her late father and sister. She also wished for a daughter to share the moment. Some months later during a conversation about women in politics, she mentioned this thought to Noeline Blackwell of the Rape Crisis Centre. Blackwell later sent the newly appointed minister a message: 'What you are doing is inspiring girls anyway.'

As Minister for Culture, Heritage and the Gaeltacht, Madigan joined one of the most exclusive clubs in Irish political life – female cabinet members. The TD for Dublin–Rathdown was very conscious that she was following in the footsteps of Countess Constance Markievicz – the country's first female minister. 'The one moment that really struck me was when I sat down at the cabinet table for the very first time and I had a moment at the table by myself. And I looked behind me on the wall and it was the

Countess Markievicz painting hanging behind me.' Madigan is very aware that she is one of four women at the cabinet table: 'It disappoints me a bit, to be honest.' She believes it would make a difference if there were more women at cabinet. On some subconscious level, she says, it must be 'a little bit daunting as a woman, when you are in the minority. Maybe in some way that actually impacts you, even though you are not really conscious of it.'

Other female ministers were particularly conscious of being a minority, especially at official events. Nora Owen recalls attending social functions as Minister for Justice in the 1994 to 1997 period where she was one of only a handful of women in the room: 'You found yourself talking to two or three men, who almost kind of gravitated towards you, talking about some policy thing or what was going on. And the women would be all sitting somewhere else. And now and again I would say, "Oh God, this isn't good". She feared they would say, "There you are, Nora, surrounded by men." It would make me feel a little bit uncomfortable, because I thought, well, what do I do? There was only such a small number of women that of necessity most of your socialising was done in male company.'

Máire Geoghegan-Quinn says this situation did not bother her, but that she was aware of it: 'It was always at the back of my mind that there would always be a comment, because even if you were only out with the head of one of the organisations that I would have been dealing with or have responsibility for, they were inevitably all male people. So you would often have a meeting and there would be just you and that person. And you would always be conscious of the fact that other people passing by would recognise you, not recognise the man that you are with, and would automatically make assumptions. And so you were conscious of that.' As a female minister, Geoghegan-Quinn was also mindful that if she made a mistake she risked letting other women down: 'If you had a cold or you had a cough – so I could identify with Theresa May when she got the fit of coughing – that was always in the back of your mind. If I'm being criticised, it's not just me personally that's being criticised, it's every female that could be in this job or that will be in this job.'

Geoghegan-Quinn felt as Minister for Justice (1993–94) she had to be seen to be tough and to lay down the law: 'There would have been nothing for the male minister to prove. He's one of us kind of thing, you know.' She says 'talking to Nora or Gemma or Mary O'Rourke or Mary Coughlan, I think they would all have experienced the same thing. Even if unconscious bias wasn't there, you always felt it was there. And you always felt that you had a huge responsibility for any other woman coming into politics, to be able to aspire to any job, including the top job. You had to be almost a trailblazer. You had to be twice as strong as any man that would do it. You had to be twice as good as any man.' She recalls one 'really bad first encounter' with one of the garda representative bodies when a member of a delegation started to shout loudly at her: 'When he stopped to take a breath, I said, "I think we will start this meeting all over again. There will be no shouting in the office. You will go outside to another office, calm yourself down and you will come in and we will do business. I don't shout at anybody. We will get much more business done by not shouting."' On another occasion, she was informed that 'a very irate man' had been on the telephone. The caller, she was told, was the garda commissioner, who was not happy that she had visited a garda station without his knowledge. A senior official told her that the commissioner wanted to pass on a message 'that your job is to be inside in the department doing legislation and doing all that stuff, and his job is out on the ground, going around'. But the commissioner was swiftly informed of the minister's likely response, 'it will be two words, tell the commissioner two words and the second one is going to be off'.

Jan O'Sullivan agrees that women have to be seen to be 'stronger' and sometimes loud when holding ministerial office: 'Some women probably do feel they have to be loud. I probably would be perceived as being fairly quiet. I think I probably have to work harder as a result of that. I have to be very sure of my ground before I will kind of be very dogmatic about something. Whereas I have seen men be very dogmatic about something that they turn out to be wrong in, but they just move on from that, and they get dogmatic about something else. You know, I think by and large women will only be dogmatic once they are pretty sure that they are right.' Mary Harney agrees that there are gender stereotypes about female politicians. As a woman, 'you are supposed to be softly, softly. And that is a disadvantage as well.' During her career, she did not fall into this category: 'There was often a perception of me that I was too hard. There's no doubt about that.' She says she would often read articles depicting her 'as tough as an old boot, whatever that means'.

When Mary Hanafin moved from the Department of Education to Social and Family Affairs in 2008 it was the beginning of difficult economic times and of budgets marked by severe public expenditure cutbacks. She believed different standards applied as she was a female minister: 'It was probably felt that you might show a bit more heart on it. I remember being in the House, [and] kind of saying, "it's with a heavy heart that I do this" kind of thing. I remember Seán Haughey saying afterwards, "Look you were the first one to actually put a bit of humanity into what was happening by just showing your emotion," that you weren't just making a policy decision, but you recognised the impact it was going to have.'

4

Madam President – At the Áras

*It's quite difficult to be first everywhere […] to go right
up to the front of a church and have a special pulpit
there for you, to be in prime seats in the National
Concert Hall, to be […] always first.*

MARY ROBINSON

Mary Robinson succeeded six men as head of state following her election to the Irish presidency in 1990. Despite the high profile that went with her daily work as president of Ireland, Robinson acknowledges the sense of isolation inherent in the role. 'It was hard. And it was lonely,' she admits. 'You learn to count particularly on your immediate family and I mean, Nick [her husband] was wonderfully supportive and very, very close friends.'

Mary McAleese, who succeeded Robinson in 1997 and served two seven-year terms as president, acknowledges that the role can occupy an 'isolated space': 'You are out ahead, there's nobody behind you, there's nobody around you who understands where you are now going. You have to be prepared to occupy that space. So I suppose, to some extent, you could call that lonely.' Like Robinson, McAleese also recognises the support of family and friends, who she says, 'wouldn't let you be lonely'. She does not associate living and working in Áras an Uachtaráin in the Phoenix Park with loneliness: 'I never found the Áras a lonely place, because there's just so much coming and going. I loved the buzz. I loved going into the office in the morning, loved hearing Bernie Carroll [a staff member] singing with her diabolical voice first thing in the morning in the kitchen.'

The elections of Mary Robinson and Mary McAleese as heads of state brought to an end the male domination of the presidency during the previous half-century. Both women pushed the limits of the office and firmly imposed their personalities on the role during their time in the Áras. As the first two Irish women to serve as president, both came under intensive scrutiny and had to deal with issues as they carved out a new pathway for Irish women in politics.

❧ ❧ ❧

Mary Robinson's election in 1990 marked a new era in Irish political life. Irish voters broke Fianna Fáil's long-standing hold on the office and in doing so they endorsed Ireland's first female president. The new head of state held views and values – not to mention a curriculum vitae as a lawyer and politician – that spoke to a more liberal and secular society. Robinson was fully aware of the various strands of historical and social change that were tied up in her election. 'I was really conscious I must walk tall, I must do it as a woman, proudly,' she says. In her acceptance speech, she acknowledged the support of women during her successful election campaign: 'It really was a very pejorative term in those days – oh, *mná na* hÉireann. So I deliberately thanked *mná na hÉireann* who instead of rocking the cradle, rocked the system.' After the formal ceremony in Dublin Castle, there was a guard of honour for the first woman to be commander-in-chief of the Defence Forces. 'I was conscious of doing it proudly and being proud of our Defence Forces. I was now Chief of the Defence Forces,' Robinson says. The symbolism of the moment became a talking point: 'The number of people, particularly in the first couple of weeks, who kept saying to me, "I cried when I saw you on the television when you inspected the guard of honour."' Later that day in the state room of Áras an Uachtaráin, Robinson remembers quietly taking in her surroundings and reflecting on her election as the country's seventh head of state: 'There was sunlight and I kept saying over and over again, I can't believe this ... and how am I going to do it, how am I going to do it well, you know.'

A great deal had changed in Ireland by 1997, when voters were again asked who they would like to be their president. New, more liberal, legislation had been introduced in areas such as contraception, divorce and homosexuality. There were more women in the workplace – although the number of female TDs remained largely unchanged during the 1990s. The themes and issues in the presidential election were different than seven years previously, especially in relation to the emphasis on gender. 'Gender just didn't come into it', Mary McAleese says about her decision to seek the presidency in 1997. Whereas Robinson spoke about '*mná na hÉireann*', McAleese focused on 'building bridges'. She defined her campaign against the backdrop of the Northern Ireland peace process. The Provisional IRA's 1994 ceasefire, which broke down in early 1996, had been restored in July 1997. With new governments in Dublin and London – led by Bertie Ahern and Tony Blair respectively – efforts were underway to kick-start talks between the main parties in Northern Ireland, although the issue of IRA decommissioning remained unresolved. All this activity was taking place alongside an election to choose Ireland's eighth head of state. 'The political moment that we were in, the social and cultural moment we were in, vis-à-vis the peace process, vis-à-vis the poor relationships north and south, poor relationships within Northern Ireland and the relatively poor relationships on the east/west flank that had been traditional, but were now melding and melting', McAleese says.

There were three presidential candidates in 1990; Robinson was the only woman. Seven years later, four of the five candidates were women – a sign that more females were not only coming forward to run for the office but that the political parties as the main gatekeepers of the nomination process were also more open to them, in part for pragmatic electoral reasons. In 1997, McAleese was nominated by Fianna Fáil and the Progressive Democrats; she ran against Mary Banotti, the Fine Gael candidate, Adi Roche, the founder of the Chernobyl Children's Project and Labour's nominee, Independent candidate Dana Rosemary Scallon, a Eurovision song contest winner, and the only man in the contest, retired garda and victims' rights campaigner Derek Nally. 'In a funny kind of way', McAleese says this dynamic 'just took the women's thing out of the equation, because it wasn't one woman going up against four men. It wasn't one woman going up against one man. It was four women going up against one man. And it was the almost normalcy of women coming to the fore in Ireland.'

Irrespective of gender, recent presidential campaigns have effectively been personality pageants that test the most politically astute and toughest candidates. In her acceptance speech, Robinson said that when she first decided to run 'the task ahead seemed daunting but straightforward enough in the quiet of my study. The tradition of easygoing elections – or indeed no elections – for the presidency seemed to promise a fairly sedate seven months.' However, at the time of her victory, she noted 'there was nothing rational or reasonable about the campaign, which developed into a barnstorming, no-holds-barred battle ...'[29]

The 1997 campaign was no less timid. McAleese's campaign came under serious criticism near the final stages of the contest. 'The attempt to smear me had nothing to do, I think, with misogyny or being a woman', she says. The threat to her candidacy emerged after leaked documents from the Department of Foreign Affairs suggested she was 'soft on Sinn Féin'. The damaging comments were written at a time when the Provisional Irish Republican Army (IRA) was not on ceasefire. The context of the accusation was even more complex. The previous year McAleese was among a handful of people invited by the Redemptorist priest Father Alec Reid to participate in private talks to promote peace in Northern Ireland following the collapse of the August 1994 IRA ceasefire. Faced with the damaging leaked document in the presidential campaign, she decided not to publicly divulge the context of her involvement: 'Why would I jeopardise something that was ultimately such benefit to the peace process just to promote my own candidacy?' With her credentials under fire and concerned about the security implications for her family, McAleese discussed her options with her husband: 'Martin and I talked it over, and I said, this is the point at which I bail out.' She decided she would inform the Fianna Fáil director of elections Noel Dempsey that she 'was going to withdraw'. But this never happened. The next morning a member of the Redemptorist Order publicly disclosed the existence of the peace initiative. This intervention, McAleese says, 'recalibrated' the debate.

On the same morning, McAleese also received an unexpected gift in the post – a pectoral cross from the sister of a priest that she had known growing up and who had since died: 'My son is called

Justin [...] and the reason he's called Justin is that in 1969 a priest who was a great mentor of mine, Father Justin Coyne, a Mullingar man, who died just as the Troubles broke out in Ardoyne, but who had been a great mentor from [when] I was about fourteen. And if you say that now, you know, in the context of priests and what have you, people's eyes will roll. But in fact, this man, more than any other human being I think in my life, helped give my life great purpose and direction.' This gift, along with the significant intervention of the Redemptorist Order, ensured McAleese got 'stuck back into the fray'. Both incidents proved pivotal in her journey to become Ireland's eighth president. McAleese later told Noel Dempsey of her decision to pull out of the campaign. 'I wouldn't like to tell you what Noel said,' she laughs, adding 'It doesn't bear repetition.' McAleese went on to win the 1997 contest and in doing so became the first woman in the world to follow another woman into the office of elected head of state.[30]

✻ ✻ ✻

Both Mary Robinson and Mary McAleese redefined and transformed the office of the president. In differing ways, they both put their own stamp and personality on the role. As academic Yvonne Galligan puts it, their elections 'herald[ed] a discernible change of pace, tone and focus in the office. The relatively staid backwater that was the received image of the Irish presidency became charged with a new political energy.'[31] As they both approached the end of their terms in office, each woman was more popular than they were on their presidential election day.[32]

On arriving at Áras an Uachtaráin, Robinson remembers resisting attempts to 'manage' her. Not long after being elected, she was presented with a legislative bill to sign. She put pen to paper and signed her name: Mary Robinson. An official took exception: 'No, no, you must sign *Máire Mhic Róibín,*' he said. The new president replied, 'Well, I don't use that as a name.' The official was not finished: 'We will come back to it, Uachtarán,' he asserted. Robinson had other thoughts. 'No, we won't come back to it,' she said to herself. Robinson sees the incident as an example of how the system failed to appreciate the changes inherent in her election. She does not think such an approach would have been made to her predecessor Patrick Hillery: 'I doubt it. I think he [the official] just thought he could manage me.'

Robinson's election brought other changes in how the Áras operated. Three security personnel were to be assigned to her at all times. She requested that 'one of them has to be a woman'. This caused a difficulty. 'Well, I'm sorry, but there's no woman trained,' the new president was told. 'What do you mean?' she asked. It emerged that there was a problem because no female officer had been trained in firearms. 'Well, train them,' Robinson said. Seven years later, when McAleese arrived in the Áras, she noticed that the vast majority of women who worked there were household staff. Drawing on her past role as an equal opportunities trainer in Queen's University, McAleese decided to address the issue. She proudly observes that 'a number of the staff, who were girls who worked in the kitchen, got master's degrees during my time there. Starting off with, you know, certificate, certificated courses, through diplomas, through degrees, through master's ...'

❖ ❖ ❖

Mary Robinson gave the presidency – which has very limited political power – a more activist role while remaining within the constitutional boundaries of the office. Her inauguration speech set the tone for how she planned to work as president: 'The Ireland

I will be representing is a new Ireland, open, tolerant, inclusive.' She also referenced 'a new, pluralist Ireland.'[33] During her seven years in office, Robinson engaged with local, community and voluntary organisations as well as opening the doors of the Áras to marginalised groups. She remembers 'wonderful visits' by members of the Traveller community to Áras an Uachtaráin: 'They had never been there before. And they would poke at things and look at things in a way that was terrific. They would make themselves feel at home.' Many visits to community groups highlighted the lack of prominence afforded to women and their achievements. She says it was normal that she would have been 'met by the man who was chair of the committee, but I would listen, and then I would learn that it was Sister Anne actually who was most responsible. And she would have been standing at the back. I would make a point of going over and shaking the hand of Sister Anne and praising her. And everybody would clap.' She feels it was a subtle but important gesture.

The role of women in the emerging peace process was also something Robinson was conscious of promoting: 'I always feel in a peace process, women are far more important than is realised, and under-represented. They are actually there on the ground making peace.' In meeting local community groups from Northern Ireland, Robinson recalls that, 'it was women who were coming out from the housing estates and linking across [communities]. The men weren't doing it, but the women were. And that it was really important to recognise that. I remember a couple of visits from women from Northern Ireland, by God, they had done themselves up to the ninety-nines. The first time in Dublin, first time in the Áras.'

Robinson's term as president spanned historic moments, such as the first IRA ceasefire in 1994 and the first Sinn Féin TD to take a seat in the Dáil in modern times in 1997. Although she visited Northern Ireland eighteen times during her presidency,[34] her trip to Belfast in June 1993 caused huge political tensions and made international headlines. She had accepted an invitation to meet various community groups, including many women's groups in west Belfast. During the visit, it was planned that she would privately meet with local politicians, including the Sinn Féin president, Gerry Adams. The inclusion of Adams was highly controversial, Robinson recalls, as the Provisional IRA, with which Sinn Féin was associated, was still engaged in a campaign of violence against the British presence in Northern Ireland. Prior to Robinson's visit, unionist politicians and the British government raised objections. Concern was also expressed in government circles in Dublin, particularly by Labour leader Dick Spring, who was Minister for Foreign Affairs in the Albert Reynolds-led Fianna Fáil–Labour coalition.

Robinson was aware of the objections to her visit: 'I had had a lot of these community people down in [Áras an Uachtaráin], and I knew that it was incredibly important that I would go [to Belfast]. And I knew that unfortunately I would also have to shake the hand of Gerry Adams. That was just the price that had to be paid.' As she recalls, the decision to go ahead with the trip – and to shake Adams's hand in private along with meeting other local representatives – heightened tensions with the Fianna Fáil–Labour government. Robinson believes that part of Spring's motivation was territorial as the peace process was part of his ministerial brief. But Robinson also thinks that she was treated differently to the previous male presidents. 'I think there was a different treatment,' she says, adding, 'Certainly Albert Reynolds was heard to remark at one stage, "She's like Ayers Rock, you move around her," you know,' she says, laughing. 'So I was quite proud of that.'

There had also been tensions with the previous Fianna Fáil-led administration headed by Charles Haughey. Following her election, in which she defeated Haughey's candidate and loyal supporter Brian Lenihan, Robinson was confronted by friction over what was understood as the remit of the presidency and her right to give media interviews. Robinson remembers one occasion, in 1991, when the government expressed concern about possible censure from China if she accepted an invitation to attend a Tibetan exhibition in the Chester Beatty Library in Dublin to be opened by the Dalai Lama. The Taoiseach made it known that the Tibetan leader should not be received in Áras an Uachtaráin nor was Robinson to meet him. When Robinson decided to accept the invitation, a stand-off ensued between the Office of the Taoiseach and the Áras. In the end, Haughey backed down. 'I mean, starting off, Charlie Haughey was not pro-me,' Robinson says, adding, 'That wasn't down to gender.' She says being a constitutional lawyer 'helped greatly' in defining the limits of how she could operate as president.

❧ ❧ ❧

By the time Mary McAleese was elected president in 1997, the idea of the occupant of Áras an Uachtaráin visiting Northern Ireland was far less controversial, despite the still uncertain peace process at that time. McAleese was the first person from Northern Ireland to become president of the Republic of Ireland. In her two terms in office she made over a hundred visits to the North on official business.[35] Members of unionist and nationalist communities from Northern Ireland were also invited to the Áras. She believes being a woman and mother was a 'big bonus' in making these visits a success as many guests did not feel 'threatened by a woman': 'When we were starting to bring people to the Áras, particularly people who were what I would call the hard-to-reach communities in Northern Ireland, I always said, we are not going to talk politics. We are not going to talk the hard stuff. We will talk the soft stuff. We just talked about families – tell me about your kids, what are they doing, where are they at in their lives, you know, have you any grandkids. People always want to talk about their kids.' Over time, trust was built up and relationships developed: 'We were bringing people to the Áras, particularly from the loyalist community and the unionist community, and bringing them back, and then bringing them back again. And building up the relationship and a network with them.' McAleese says she adopted a team approach with her husband, Martin. He would make initial contact with different groups and over time he gained 'huge respect' from the leaders of these groups for these efforts. 'For these kind of macho, male-dominated cohorts,' she says 'the first person they engaged with was Martin rather than me. They would meet me eventually, but he was the conduit to me.' When the meetings eventually took place, 'they had a huge respect for the presidency, huge respect for the role of the president'.

McAleese thinks that shared motherhood experiences also facilitated bonding with other visitors, most notably the British head of state, Queen Elizabeth II. She believes the fact 'we were two mammies' was helpful. They talked 'about what we could do as, as mothers to change the course of history for the children of other mothers to come'. McAleese says Queen Elizabeth and 'her family had been really badly hit by Lord Mountbatten's death. We had those things in common. I also had been very badly hit by deaths that had touched us personally. We were not at all inhibited about discussing those things.'

The first meeting between an Irish president and a British monarch took place in 1993, when Mary Robinson travelled to Buckingham Palace. Robinson says she was conscious of the symbolic nature of this visit, that it was a moment of history. She recalls the national anthem, *Amhrán na bhFiann*, being played during her visit. Among the topics discussed by the Irish president and Queen Elizabeth II was their shared interest in horses. When Robinson raised the prospect of the queen visiting Ireland in the future, she says '[the queen's] face lit up and she responded warmly. It was quite obvious that was something she was interested in doing.'[36]

Robinson's visit was an important step in a new phase in Anglo-Irish relations as the peace process developed. During McAleese's second term in office, relations developed further with Queen Elizabeth II's state visit to Ireland in 2011. McAleese says their conversations 'were always mother-to-mother, woman to woman.' They often spoke about their children. As they were driven through Dublin, the British head of state inquired about one of McAleese's daughters who had recently married. The queen asked, 'How are the young marrieds getting on?' 'Great,' McAleese replied. The queen then enquired, 'Did they do what they all do now, did they live together beforehand?' 'Certainly not,' McAleese answered. 'How come?' the queen asked. 'Well, two reasons,' the president explained, 'I would have killed her and his mother would have killed him.' As the queen heard this explanation, McAleese recalls, 'she just started to laugh'.

❧ ❧ ❧

As the elected heads of state, both Mary Robinson and Mary McAleese became public personalities. The position of president required them to be constantly in the spotlight. For their families, there were unintended practical consequences.

Robinson's three children were born in the early stages of a busy political life that co-existed with her developing legal career.

She was first elected to the Seanad in 1969, the beginning of a 20-year career as a senator. She ran for the Dáil twice, in 1977 and 1981, unsuccessfully on both occasions. She was also a member of Dublin City Council from 1979 to 1983.

'Tessa was born in 1972, William was born in 1974 and Aubrey was born at the time of the general election in 1981,' she says. Of all Robinson's political and legal activities, her bid for the presidency in 1990 had the biggest effect on family life: 'The impact on the children was quite significant, because we had kept them very, very private. I mean, even though I had been a senator for twenty years, there was no photograph of me and Nick with the children in the public domain.' During the presidential campaign, they had a photograph taken of the family for a national newspaper: 'We put the dog in as well. Nick and myself are smiling in our political way and the three children in the middle have the most grim faces and even the dog had a grim face. It was a very funny photograph.'

On the night of her election as president, Robinson spoke with her children about the implications of her elevation. She recalls 'saying over and over again, "Even though I'm now going to be president of Ireland, you matter more to me than anything else."' She tried to make the Áras as much of a family home as possible: 'We had our quarters upstairs, and the only person who could come upstairs was somebody who had been looking after us in our home, who was allowed to come and work with us in the Áras. So we knew her already.'

During her time in the Áras, she remembers her children were 'very solicitous of the light in the window'. As a symbolic gesture, Robinson placed a light in an upstairs window of Áras an Uachtaráin to mark the welcome Ireland extends to Irish emigrants and their descendants. She remembers her children's reaction to the newly introduced tradition: 'That was really important. And I remember one night and I think it was the only time it happened – the Áras was affected by a blackout and Aubrey actually went and put a candle in the window.'

Robinson remembers frequent reminders that the Áras was a home as well as the residence of the head of state: 'At an early stage, we had a party for Aubrey's friends from school. And they played a game of putting messages on chairs, hide-and-seek basically. I remember coming in for a formal meeting with an ambassador the following day and there was a note still on the chair. It wasn't rude luckily. But it was just funny, you know.'

The Robinsons made an effort to ensure their children felt at home in the Áras. She recalls her son later 'had drums in a room down at the far end' where she adds 'he could bang away as much as he wanted'. But she admits the seven years of her presidential term were hard on her children. By way of an example she mentions when her son Aubrey was playing soccer for his national school: 'He cut himself. And there was a photographer there, and he took a photograph of Aubrey, the bloodied face, and it was [in the newspapers].' When he went to secondary school, he had to be taken by car. She remembers that he always insisted at being dropped around the corner so, she says, 'he could walk to school'. There were also hassles when her older children tried to get a taxi back to the Áras. 'Getting into a taxi and saying, "Take me to Áras an Uachtaráin" [and the reply] "Oh feck off, you little …",' she laughs.

Robinson also noticed that during this time her 'children didn't really make new friends. They deepened the friendship with their existing friends, and were very slow to make new friends.' When her eldest son, William, was a university student in Scotland, she announced she was leaving the Áras in 1997. The story was reported on television in Scotland. William had just moved into new accommodation and one of his new flatmates asked about his surname and if he was related to the departing

Irish president. William's reply was somewhat evasive. The new flatmate asked another question: 'What do your parents do for a living?' As Robinson recalls, 'As quick as a flash, William said, "they are between jobs".'

McAleese's son Justin was equally evasive about his parents' identities. She recalls that when he first met his future husband, Fionán Donohoe, he said he was a 'distant' relative of the Irish president. Several meetings later, when they were discussing their families, he revealed his mother was called Mary and his father Martin. The penny dropped.

When McAleese was elected as Ireland's second female president in 1997, the move to the Áras also involved major adaption for her children: 'The twins were thirteen and Emma was fifteen. They did not know what it meant. It hadn't really occurred to them that within minutes they would be moving to live in Dublin.' The family had been living in Rostrevor in Co. Down: 'We lived in the middle of the village, in front of the post office, beside the church, around the corner from their primary school, a bus ride away from their second-level school. They knew everybody. They couldn't put their nose out the door without being related to somebody. That's a very different environment from moving into the heartland of the Phoenix Park, where no bus passes the front door.' The children had to enrol in new schools. 'Poor Emma was parachuted into Junior Cert year. I don't know how she coped with that,' McAleese recalls. Her other daughter Sara also had to adjust. 'She really just took Martin and I on, what kind of school were we after sending her to, that they didn't play camogie. She was horrified.'

McAleese says the fact that her father-in-law lived with them helped to 'created a little space in the Áras that was our home'. They initially lived 'above the shop' in the Áras. But due to 'an asbestos problem', the family moved to another area in the building away from the offices and official reception rooms: 'It meant then that we could colonise a place as far away as humanly possible from what I would call the official buzz of the Áras.' There were other practical advantages: 'More importantly we could have a door that my children were not bringing their muddy boots and their bicycles through, because at one point they were bringing them through the main front door of the Áras. And I just couldn't be having that. You know, kicking off their boots in the front hall. No, thank you very much.'

As with the Robinsons, there were practical issues that had to be addressed in the move into the Áras. Security advice recommended garda drivers for the children. 'We weren't able to dictate what happened. We were told what happened,' McAleese says. Even before they moved into the Áras, the family had to deal with security issues arising from the controversy over leaked documents suggesting McAleese was soft on Sinn Féin. 'The immediate impact on my family was atrocious,' she recalls. 'Bear in mind, this was 1997, all forms of paramilitarism were still strongly active. My children were at school in Kilkeel. Immediately the flag went up about their safety. That was devastating.' During her presidency, she says they were always mindful of the 'security implications'. There were 'worrying ones over the years that we simply were not in a position to discuss publicly. But we had to always protect our children.'

5

SEXISM
– #POLITICIANSTOO

I felt a chuck on my bra strap at the back. I got a shock …

GEMMA HUSSEY

Gemma Hussey was a member of Seanad Éireann when she had an unsettling experience in Leinster House. She was sponsoring a private members bill on rape. She had walked across from the Seanad to observe a debate in the Dáil: 'I was sitting on the edge of the Dáil chamber. There's a circle that goes around above the chamber, where senators sit to observe Dáil debates. And I was sitting there observing a debate when I felt a chuck on my bra strap at the back. I got a shock and I leapt to my feet.'

When Hussey turned around, she was face to face with Charles Haughey, who had recently been elected Fianna Fáil leader and Taoiseach. 'He kind of gestured to me to sit down,' Hussey recalls. 'I just wanted to say to you, Senator – don't worry about your bill,' Haughey advised. 'We will look after your bill because I have an excellent minister who will steer it through, Mr Seán Doherty.' Hussey was still struggling for words as Haughey departed:

'I was dumbfounded. I was just amazed. I was kind of rendered speechless, really.'

Today, such behaviour could be considered a resigning matter. In any workplace, such inappropriate behaviour would automatically trigger a formal response and disciplinary action. This incident would not be out of place in the revelations arising from the #metoo movement in the second decade of the 21st century. Women, particularly those in the public sphere, are coming forward to tell their stories. The incident above took place almost forty years ago, in the national parliament. It was never raised or remedied.

This incident was not Hussey's first uncomfortable encounter with Haughey. She recalls what she describes as 'a strange incident' in the late 1970s when the Fianna Fáil politician was Minister for Health. Haughey was introducing legislation to liberalise the availability of contraception. But many people, including Hussey, were critical of what they saw as the restrictive nature of the legislation, which required a doctor's prescription to obtain contraception for family planning purposes – essentially limiting availability to married couples.

Hussey sought a meeting with the Minister for Health to press for changes to the government's proposals. She had not met Haughey previously: 'I was sent a message that the Minister for Health would see me. So I found his office and I went in.' Haughey was with one of his department officials. He introduced himself: 'Hello Gemma. How are you?'

Hussey was surprised at the informality: 'I took a bit of umbrage because I had been very formal and called him Minister.' He duly dismissed the civil servant and Hussey outlined why she considered the legislation too conservative: 'He listened and then he looked at me and kind of silence fell and he looked at me across the table. "Well, Gemma," he said, "I don't need to tell you that the

Billings method (a method of natural family planning) doesn't suit me any more than it would suit you." The Wicklow politician was left flummoxed by the outrageous remark: 'My breath was taken away. I didn't know where to look. I muttered something about, "Well, I just came to tell you my views." And I stumbled out of the room.'

These are not the only inappropriate incidents that Hussey had to deal with in her political career. At the end of 1982, Garret FitzGerald appointed Hussey – by now a TD – as Minister for Education in his Fine Gael–Labour coalition. She was the first woman to hold this position. The job required attending teacher union conferences every Easter. On one occasion, Hussey was speaking with a union leader when a drunken teacher approached: 'He came from behind me and groped me, my bosom, you know, put his two hands down and started feeling me up. I leapt to my feet, and I said to the fella beside me, "I'm going to my room." I was just disgusted, and I was angry.' Several union executives subsequently expressed regret at the incident, but the man who had behaved so inappropriately never apologised to the Minister for Education. Today there would be an expectation that such behaviour, witnessed by many, would lead to disciplinary action at a minimum.

Hussey is not the only female politician who has had to deal with this type of offensive behaviour. A female colleague confided in her about 'a serious grope' in a lift in Leinster House: 'The thing about it was that the fella who did it was a "Holy Joe". He was one of the people, you know, against contraception, against divorce, against everything else. But that's not why it happened. It was because he was just an old lecher and he was a hypocrite.'

Former Minister for Justice Nora Owen admits that among the male politicians she encountered in Leinster House, there were 'probably one or two that you wouldn't feel overly comfortable getting into the lift with'. But reflecting in general on her time as a Fine Gael TD, Owen says most politicians were fairly respectful of each other. Had a male colleague ever acted inappropriately towards her, Owen says she would 'probably just tell them to eff-off or something'. Such an up-front approach would also have been favoured by Mary Coughlan, who was a Fianna Fáil cabinet minister from 2002 to 2011: 'If somebody did something in my view that wasn't appropriate, as in touch or something like that, I would just let them know that I was going to end up better off than them when we were finished.'

Labour's Niamh Bhreathnach was less fortunate during the five years she spent in Leinster House from 1992 to 1997. Bhreathnach had to deal with several physical incidents, which she attributes to 'macho bullying'. On one occasion during voting in the Dáil chamber, a male opposition politician, who she describes as 'quite drunk', approached her to make a representation about a constituency matter. Bhreathnach, who was Minister for Education, was unable to assist with the request. Her response was met with, 'Listen here, you.' She says the TD then started shoving her with his arm and she banged her head against the wall: 'There was a lovely Malton print behind me, and I did wonder did I crack the glass but evidently I didn't.' She confided in a colleague about what had happened: 'I was told, "Look, forget about that, he won't remember it in the morning."' Decades later, she, however, has not forgotten it.

On another occasion, Bhreathnach recalls being elbowed by two male opposition politicians as she was walking to the Dáil chamber to vote: 'We were going down and the bells were ringing. I thought in the beginning they were being funny. And then I realised they weren't.' Both politicians were opposed to education changes being introduced by Bhreathnach. 'It was like being out in the school yard,' the teacher-turned-minister says. 'Don't forget,

I had taught boys. And it was that kind of physical behaviour. It wasn't directed at me, you see, as a woman. If I was a man, they would probably have done the very same.'

The issue of 'male power' or 'male dominance' is never far away when many of the female ministers discuss their experiences of working in Leinster House. And such attitudes were not always confined to elected representatives. In the mid-1980s, Máire Geoghegan-Quinn was a Fianna Fáil member of the Oireachtas Committee on Marriage Breakdown. As part of the committee's work, the members met the Knights of Columbanus, a male-only lay Catholic organisation. As Geoghegan-Quinn recalls, 'They came in and they had a document. And on every page of the document, you had a man's hand on top of a woman's. That was not something that happened [by] coincidence, you know. This was very deliberate.' The Galway West TD asked: 'Is there a reason why on every single page, the male hand is on top of the female hand?' She says it was 'a very kind of innocent in a way question'. The response of one of the representatives was not what she had expected: 'He turned on me and he read the riot act. He finished it up by saying, "and by the way, I would remind Deputy Geoghegan-Quinn that the largest number of members of our organisation outside of Dublin are in her constituency".' Before Geoghegan-Quinn had an opportunity to respond, her Fianna Fáil colleague and fellow committee member Pádraig Flynn 'went through him like a dose of salts. Pádraig just jumped in, and he said, "Are you threatening my colleague?"'

The same Pádraig Flynn was in the spotlight for less benign reasons in the latter part of the presidential election campaign in 1990. A comment during a discussion on RTÉ Radio 1 by the Fianna Fáil minister shocked many of his party colleagues, outraged large swathes of voters and created an upswing of support for the campaign of Mary Robinson to the detriment of Flynn's preferred candidate, Brian Lenihan. During the radio show, Flynn accused Robinson of having 'a new-found interest in family, being a mother, and all that kind of thing'. For good measure, he added that 'none of us who knew Mary Robinson very well in previous incarnations ever heard her claiming to be a great wife and mother'. Robinson was canvassing on Grafton Street in Dublin city centre when Flynn was speaking on radio: 'We had been marching up and down Grafton Street with a number of celebrities and actors, who were very supportive. And I got taken aside to say there's been this terrible interview with Pádraig Flynn.' From a campaign perspective, the timing proved important. 'Pádraig Flynn had done me a huge favour,' Robinson pragmatically admits.

The effect was immediately noticeable in Niamh Bhreathnach's Dún Laoghaire constituency, where Bhreathnach was organising a canvass for Robinson later the same afternoon. 'I actually heard the radio show at home,' she says, adding 'people had promised to canvass. But so many [more] people came, I actually had to send them to Booterstown and Monkstown.'

The impact of Flynn's comment was also recognised in Lenihan's campaign. His sister Mary O'Rourke remembers listening to Flynn's comments on the radio, and thinking, 'Oh, my God. OH, MY GOD.' After a rocky few weeks in the presidential election, O'Rourke had believed her brother's campaign was heading towards victory. But the negative impact of the interview was immediate and crucial: 'By the time I did the canvassing in Tyrrellspass and came home that night, it was everywhere.' Beyond political ties and sibling loyalty, O'Rourke retains a harsh view of the remarks from another perspective: 'How dare he. Sure, she would have always had an interest in her clothes and her family.'

Another senior Fianna Fáil female politician had a similar response: 'I died. I died. I died. I was so embarrassed. Oh, God Almighty. I could have killed him. I could have killed him,'

Máire Geoghegan-Quinn admits. While Flynn 'kind of poo-pooed at the beginning', Geoghegan-Quinn says 'at the back of his mind, he's too intelligent not to know what an impact that had'. She remembers that, 'there wasn't one person in the parliamentary party that didn't say it to him at the time'.

❧ ❧ ❧

Being subjected to dismissive sexist remarks is something many female politicians have experienced. In 1992, Taoiseach Albert Reynolds famously brushed off Nora Owen's interruptions during heated Dáil exchanges by saying 'that's women for ya'. Reflecting on the exchange, Owen says, 'It was a sexist remark. A lot of men interrupted him and he didn't say, "That's men for you".' Owen's criticism is, however, somewhat muted: 'I'm sad that it was Albert. I don't think he was sexist and, to be honest, I think he was a polite courteous man and would have opened doors and stood up and given a woman a seat. He was that kind of courteous man. So I don't think he was being sexist. He really wanted to say, "Would you shut up and listen to me?" but he didn't. He said, "You are not listening, and that's women for you."'

Several years after the infamous incident, one of Reynolds's five daughters told Owen how the family had responded: 'She said, "Oh, we were all very cross with our dad for saying that." Because they were all very modern women.' Máire Geoghegan-Quinn, a close political ally of Reynolds, also raised the controversy with him at the time: 'I had a go at him and I said, you never say that, ever again.' He replied to her: 'I shouldn't have said that. I know that.' Like Owen, Geoghegan-Quinn describes Reynolds as 'a gentleman'. She says 'he was surrounded by the strongest women especially Kathleen [Reynolds's wife] and his daughters. I mean, anybody that knows them, would say, by God, he wouldn't get away with that at home.'

As Minister for Justice in the Rainbow Coalition from 1994 to 1997, Nora Owen faced constant fire from John O'Donoghue, Fianna Fáil's justice spokesperson. Their exchanges in the Dáil chamber were stormy and combative in a period that included a siege in Mountjoy Jail and high-profile gangland criminal activity, including the murder of journalist Veronica Guerin. With justice matters dominating the daily headlines, Mary O'Rourke admits Owen had a 'tough time'. Observing from the Fianna Fáil side of the Dáil, O'Rourke recalls occasionally thinking 'God, John, that was rough, wasn't it?' When she relayed her concerns to O'Donoghue, he merely replied, 'Part of the game, Mary, part of the game'. O'Rourke admired Owen's steely determination, but she says many other women have shared similar experiences: 'People like to have a scapegoat. Don't they? And sometimes a woman fits the bill for a scapegoat.'

Interestingly, another Fianna Fáil politician holds a different view on O'Donoghue's approach. Mary Hanafin was familiar with the Fianna Fáil strategy as her husband Eamon Leahy was a key advisor to O'Donoghue: 'Eamon wrote John O'Donoghue's speeches and things like that. So I knew exactly where that was coming from. So I took a particular pleasure not at him knocking Nora [but] in him winning the argument with a really good speech.'

The female minister who was being targeted, Owen, saw these interactions with her Fianna Fáil counterpart as 'the cut and thrust' of political debate: 'I think John O'Donoghue recognised that you know, I wasn't going to be able to do an awful lot about some of the crime and that there wasn't enough money around to do it. He was just relentless and he loved the media coverage. You know, he really gave good copy.' She admits, however, that the exchanges took their toll: 'When I would leave the chamber, I would be shaking sometimes [after] the onslaught. Because it was an onslaught, you know.' Notwithstanding the ferocity of these exchanges, the two political adversaries actually got on well outside the Dáil chamber: 'Off camera he was very nice to me actually. I would meet him and say, "You were in fine form today, John." And he would say, "Oh, honest to God, you remind me of my mother." His mother was a widow and she had to fight very hard for her children and everything. And he said, "You are as tough as she is." Because I never gave in to him.'

Owen believes O'Donoghue would have adopted the same approach had he been facing a male minister heading up the Department of Justice during the life of the Rainbow Coalition. And while she does not believe O'Donoghue adopted a sexist approach towards her, she thinks that the fact that she was a woman heightened interest in the exchanges with other politicians and the media: 'It made better copy that I was a woman minister because I think it looked as if he was battering me down. Although when I re-read some of the Dáil debates I'm very pleased with the way I reacted.'

❖ ❖ ❖

In November 2010, the reaction of Taoiseach Brian Cowen to heckling from Labour's Joan Burton resulted in him apologising for a remark widely viewed as sexist. During tetchy exchanges during the economic crisis in the Dáil, Fianna Fáil's Cowen did not take kindly to Burton's interjections. Addressing Labour leader Eamon Gilmore, Cowen asked could he 'try and rein her in now and again'. Burton says the remark 'was absolutely sexist in its expression. I don't think in a million years he would have said that to a man.' Burton singles out male politicians including Noël

Browne, Dick Spring and Mervyn Taylor as mentors when she first embarked on a political career in the late 1980s. She first won a Dáil seat in 1992. Her experience of some other male politicians has, however, been defined by 'roaring and shouting and being quite abusive'. Many female politicians, Burton believes, have also experienced what she describes as 'man rage'.

With the advent of social media in recent years, comments in the Dáil and Seanad chambers viewed as inappropriate are generally called out with more immediate public and media reaction. During the 2013 referendum campaign to abolish the Seanad, David Norris accused Regina Doherty of Fine Gael of 'talking through her fanny'. The Trinity College senator also described Doherty's comments about Seanad abolition as 'the Regina monologue'. Doherty was a first-time TD, having been elected in the 2011 general election, and was her party's deputy director of elections for the referendum campaign. Norris subsequently said he regretted if his comments had caused any offence. He said he was 'very happy to withdraw' the remarks, which he said had been made 'off the top of my head'. He accepted his language had been 'intemperate'.[37] 'So like, he said he regretted saying it, but he wasn't sorry he said it,' Doherty says. In her view what Norris said 'patently is sexist'. She says, 'I think he thought he was being funny. He was seriously undermined and threatened by the fact that I was involved in the referendum.' She adds, 'He was just an eejit.' She has moved on, she says and there are no hard feelings: 'God, no.'

Mary Hanafin also harbours no ill will about comments made by colleagues when she was being appointed Government Chief Whip in 2002. She was the first woman to hold the position. The move attracted a lot of remarks from some of her colleagues. 'The number of people who at the time said to me, "Well, it's the first time I have been whipped by a woman,"' Hanafin recalls.

'It wasn't meant to be sexist. I didn't take it as sexist. I think they were trying to make light of the fact that I wasn't in the cabinet.'

Nora Owen says the most sexist remark she experienced during her ministerial career came not from a fellow politician but from a journalist. Following a controversy in the justice area, a reporter mused that the situation would have been different – and better – had Michael Noonan, Owen's Fine Gael colleague, been Minister for Justice. The point being made was that the Department of Justice job wasn't 'really a role for women', Owen believes. 'I remember being very angry about it. And then just saying, well, it was just a stupid thing to say. I said, can you imagine the criminals sitting around deciding whether they would commit a crime because a male or a female minister was in charge?'

Another female minister also took issue with media commentary. In the 1980s, Máire Geoghegan-Quinn remembers chairing an Oireachtas committee that was examining women's issues, including the characterisation of women in the media: 'In those days, you would have the women, you know, loving her clothes because it was so white and she wanted it to be even whiter. And then you had the woman draped over a tractor or a car being sold.' The committee sought the views of several national newspaper editors on the appropriateness of this type of coverage and advertising. One editor, Geoghegan-Quinn recalls, 'sent us a letter, basically, giving us the two fingers'. His view was that 'a woman draped over an article for sale, or a tractor or a car or whatever, was infinitely more pleasing to the eye than a male would be. And that incensed every member of the committee.' So when it came to the publication of the committee's report, the members decided to include the letter. 'I'm told he was livid,' the former Galway politician muses.

On a more personal note, Mary O'Rourke still recalls the comment of one journalist when she lost her Dáil seat in the 2002 general election. O'Rourke was an outgoing minister and deputy leader of Fianna Fáil. During a live television interview as the election results were being discussed, a male journalist suggested to her, 'I suppose you will be back to your knitting.' O'Rourke says she never knitted. She also never forgot the remark: 'I haven't forgotten it, no. I haven't.' As the recent high-profile example of Hillary Clinton demonstrates, such remarks are not confined to Ireland or the past. In December 2017, a spokeswoman for *Vanity Fair* magazine had to apologise after it published a 'humorous' video suggesting the former United States presidential candidate should 'take up knitting' rather than run for office again.[38]

❧ ❧ ❧

The number of recorded incidents in Irish political life involving unwarranted physical approaches is relatively low although a handful have garnered significant public notoriety. In 1998, there was an incident involving a Fianna Fáil TD, Liam Aylward and a female usher outside the Dáil bar. Following a complaint, the Oireachtas authorities carried out an investigation. 'I have apologised for the incident personally and the apology was graciously accepted. I have nothing further to add,' Aylward said at the time.[39] It was reported in the media that the 'Dáil authorities now realise that the four female ushers are vulnerable to incident with TDs. Rota bosses are now considering putting them on earlier duties.'[40]

Another Fianna Fáil TD, Ned O'Keeffe, had, a number of years previous, been obliged to apologise for his behaviour following an incident in the Dáil bar in 1991 with RTÉ political correspondent Úna Claffey.[41] More recently, Tom Barry, a Fine Gael TD, had to apologise for pulling his party colleague Áine Collins onto his lap in the Dáil chamber. The incident in 2013 was captured on

Oireachtas TV and was labelled 'Lapgate' by the media after a clip of the incident was widely viewed on the internet. Barry rejected accusations that he was sexist, although the timing of the incident was embarrassing – it happened during the Dáil debate on the Protection of Life during Pregnancy Bill.[42]

Regina Doherty admits that female politicians are regrettably subjected to unwarranted attention from male colleagues. The attention often takes the form of unwanted comments, she stresses: 'There are certain men in all organisations, and it isn't unique to here [Leinster House], that think they are God's gift to women and think they only have to flutter their eyelashes or say something particularly sexual or crude to you, and you are supposed to fall down on your ground – "Oh, woe is me. I'm so lucky." There's a number of people around here that are like that. They fancy themselves something rotten and think, you know, they would have displayed amorous charms and I'm using that word very, very loosely towards people that it would have been unwanted, unwarranted ... And I suppose it doesn't stop them. That's just the way they are.'

Reflecting on a career in national politics that started in 1992, Fine Gael's Frances Fitzgerald thinks there is less sexism in Leinster House today than previously. She believes comments and remarks uttered in the past would be viewed as unacceptable in more recent times: 'The place is much more respectful and people are much more aware of issues around sexual harassment, inappropriate talk and so on. I would certainly have seen the changes in here.' As a first-time TD in 1992, she recalls, 'there was always one or two people who were sexually crude'. On one occasion, she was left shocked when one government minister made an inappropriate remark to her when she was a Fine Gael opposition spokesperson in the 1990s. The comment – 'a very crude personal remark' – was made privately in the Dáil chamber.

As she walked away, Fitzgerald replied to the minister, 'That's totally inappropriate.' While Fitzgerald believes that there was a 'generational' element involved, the incident was not forgotten by either individual. Many years later, when Fitzgerald was herself a government minister, the man in question raised the earlier exchange: 'The person approached me and said, "I'm very embarrassed about what I said to you. And I want to apologise."' Like many other women, Fitzgerald did not do anything about the incident at the time: 'I just dealt with it myself. And I think now probably if the same things happened, you probably would act on them differently.'

'You know what?' Fine Gael's Mary Mitchell O'Connor says, 'Every single woman, I believe, has experienced it somewhere along the line.' Mitchell O'Connor, who first entered the Dáil in 2011, recalls one particularly inappropriate comment that was made in her company in Leinster House: 'I actually couldn't repeat what he said. It was so disgusting. And he said it in the company of other TDs.' She adds, 'I would hate my mother or anyone that I know to think that some individual would say that to a woman.'

❧ ❧ ❧

Mary McAleese's experience of being treated differently as a female president arose outside the Irish political realm. 'The only misogyny I ever experienced as president came directly from the highest levels of the Catholic Church. I experienced it from Cardinal Law. It was highly offensive. I [also] experienced it directly from Pope John Paul II. It was highly offensive, and intended.' McAleese was on a visit to Italy and the Vatican in February 1999 when she was invited to meet Pope John Paul II. She vividly recalls being introduced to the Polish pontiff and his response: 'He ignored me. He reached right across to my husband, and he shook his hand, and he said, "Would you not prefer to be the president of Ireland instead of your wife?" And then a big laugh. He obviously thought this was incredibly funny.' No one else in the room joined in the laughter. 'He realised that nobody else thought it was funny, because, at that point, my husband was mortified. I reached across and I took his [the pope's] hand, and I said, "Holy Father, let me introduce myself. I'm the person that you are here to meet. My name is Mary McAleese. I'm the elected president of Ireland. I'm the elected president, whether you like it or whether you don't."' Sensing the annoyance of his Irish visitor, the pope duly sought to explain his behaviour. 'Oh, this was supposed to be a joke. My English is not so good,' he said, adding, 'I heard you had a great sense of humour.' McAleese replied, 'Yeah, not on this subject.' Pope John Paul II promptly issued the first of several apologies: 'He knew by my face that I didn't think it was a funny. I did say to him, "You would never have done that to a male president."' The two heads of state 'parted friends', notwithstanding McAleese's view that the pope's initial actions had been 'highly misogynistic'.

The Irish head of state did not, however, part on such friendly terms with another Catholic Church leader who, she says, was 'exceptionally rude' when they met. McAleese was on an official visit to the United States in 1998 when she met the late Cardinal Bernard Law, the Archbishop of Boston. Four years later, Law resigned from that position following accusations that he had covered up the sexual abuse of children by priests.

Back in 1998, Law was determined to discuss one particular issue with McAleese: 'He raised the issue of women priests, which I, of course, had not raised publicly as president.' Law was, however, familiar with the views McAleese had expressed on women priests prior to her election as president in 1997. The Irish delegation, which included Liz O'Donnell as a minister of state, was visiting

Law in his Boston residence. The official brief included thanking the cardinal for his efforts with Irish immigrants in Boston. As the meeting drew to a close, Law invited McAleese into an adjoining room where Mary Ann Glendon, a well-known conservative Catholic academic, was waiting.

Law proceeded to reprimand McAleese: 'He said to me in a very patronising tone of voice, "Madam, you will listen while Professor Glendon explains why women priests are simply not possible."' McAleese, however, stood her ground: 'I said to him, "Under no circumstances. I didn't come here to be lectured to by Professor Mary Ann Glendon. I came here to thank you for what you have done, and I have done that. And I regard this as completely inappropriate."' As he had raised the issue, McAleese outlined her own views on women priests. In response, Law told McAleese, 'that he was sorry for Ireland, that he was sorry that Catholic Ireland had such a terrible person as president'.

Before parting, Law also admonished Liz O'Donnell for sending her children to a Protestant school. He did not appear to be aware that McAleese's son was also enrolled in a Protestant school at the time. The meeting deteriorated further as McAleese said: 'If you think for one minute I'm going to sit here and be insulted by you on behalf of the Irish people, you have another thing coming.' She then continued, 'I have no respect for your views on women priests. I regard them as misogynistic. I regard them as theological twaddle. And now I'm telling you that.' With that exchange, Cardinal Law found out that McAleese was no pushover.

6

MEDIA AND APPEARANCE – LOOKING GREAT BUT WHAT DID SHE SAY?

On a personal level, I felt quite daunted, especially on my first day. You literally wonder where you have to go, what you have to say [and], as a woman, what to wear.

SÍLE DE VALERA

Most of the female ministers share the sentiments of Fianna Fáil's Síle de Valera. While there's an acceptance that how you look is part of the job, many believe it attracts far too much focus and commentary. Several have been subjected to particularly personal and cruel comments about how they look or what they wear. While some of their male counterparts have received similar treatment, the female cabinet members believe that has not occurred to the same extent. Some of them note that the focus on appearance might be off-putting for women who are interested in pursuing a career in political life.

De Valera still remembers what she wore when she first arrived at Leinster House in 1977. She opted for a simple summer dress: 'I didn't go looking for anything special. That dress happened to be in the wardrobe and that was what I wore.' Twenty years later, when de Valera was appointed Minister for the Arts, Heritage, Gaeltacht and the Islands, she was constantly in the spotlight and her appearance came under greater scrutiny.

One particular aspect of the heightened attention as a cabinet minister was, however, upsetting for the long-time Fianna Fáil politician: 'There was constant comments about my weight and there were comments that were very unflattering,' she says. 'I remember reading in a national newspaper – it was the beginning of the year and everyone was talking about their New Year's resolutions. And this female journalist referred to different people and what they should do. And under my name she had, "Síle should resolve to rid herself of some of her chins." I remember that being very personal and hurtful.'

De Valera left cabinet in 2002. As a consolation, Taoiseach Bertie Ahern offered her a junior ministry, which she accepted. She opted out of political life at the subsequent general election in 2007. Before her retirement, she remembers one newspaper featured an unflattering cartoon, which caused her considerable upset. 'Now, I know I am overweight but it was of this gross woman pertaining to be me,' she recalls. After seeing the unflattering cartoon, de Valera spoke to the newspaper editor: 'I said, "When you are doing the next cartoon, could you ever manage to divest me of some of my chins or some of the weight?"' Confronted in this way, the editor was, de Valera says, 'very contrite'. He replied, 'Oh Síle, I apologise about that. We never had such [a] bad reaction to anything as we did to that cartoon.'

During her political career, the former Fianna Fáil minister says she was able to block out most of these offensive remarks, but she admits this type of coverage was hurtful: 'I mean, if anyone said that to you on a personal level, it would be bad enough. But to have that magnified by way of [a] newspaper, it is even more hurtful. Because it's so public.' She is of the firm view that double standards were applied: 'There might have been a few male colleagues that mightn't have been too slim because they might have had one or two Guinness too many. [But] that was never commented on, and rightly so. But it shouldn't be commented on women either. Those sort of personal remarks should not have a place either in the working world, of which politics is a part.' Looking back on this type of coverage, de Valera believes it ultimately put many women off becoming involved in political life.

Gemma Hussey, who was a national political figure from the late 1970s until she left Dáil Éireann in 1989, shares similar views about appearance and weight. 'I was always conscious of the fact that I was overweight,' the former Fine Gael Minister for Education says. She admits that had someone commented on her weight, it would have left her devastated. When US President Ronald Reagan visited Ireland in 1984, Hussey felt under pressure about what to wear for the presidential visit: 'I took an awful lot of trouble over an outfit that I was going to wear when Reagan was over.' Eventually, she opted to get 'a dressmaker to make something for me, because I was so plump. I mostly couldn't buy off the peg.'

The subject of weight and female politicians was to the fore when Mary Hanafin once attended a Christmas pantomime of all things. During the show, she heard the actors make a joke at the expense of the Progressive Democrats leader and Tánaiste Mary Harney, her cabinet colleague. 'She doesn't know this now, but there was a comment in a pantomime about her weight,' Hanafin recalls. She clearly did not find it funny or appropriate as the next day the Fianna Fáil politician phoned the theatre to lodge a complaint: 'I contacted them and said that that was completely unnecessary. They took it out.'

When confronted by offensive remarks, especially about her appearance, Harney developed 'a thick neck' during a political career that stretched from 1977 to 2011. She opted not to follow up on negative newspaper articles about her weight or appearance: 'I think when you are very young, it might affect you. But when you are older, no.' The impact, she says, is often greatest on immediate family: 'They have a terrible effect sometimes on people's children. The people who would get more hurt about stuff in the media would be my family and my parents, in particular. My mother used to get so upset. And that would upset me.' She made efforts to avoid that happening: 'Sometimes I would say, "Don't let Mummy see that", you know.' Reflecting on the impact of social media coverage on political life in more recent times, Harney says she 'would hate to be around now with all the social media stuff and the awful things they say about people'.

Ignoring media commentary has sometimes been easier said than done. Harney recalls the reaction of her Progressive Democrats colleague Liz O'Donnell to a tabloid headline describing her as a 'blonde bombshell'. Harney says, 'She came into me and she was absolutely devastated. She was really upset, very tearful.' She says O'Donnell feared the commentary would undermine her political credibility. 'I'm not being taken seriously. How would you feel if they said that about you?' she asked her party leader. Harney replied, 'I would be thrilled.' Despite the humour involved, Harney accepted this type of media commentary should not have happened but says throughout her political career: 'You just accepted it, got on with it.' She devised a coping mechanism, which had been adopted by a former British prime minister: 'I had a habit and I learned from Margaret Thatcher – if you had a bad week, don't read the papers on Sunday. Maybe you read them a week later but just try and get your head clear. That was how I dealt with issues.'

Harney found herself at the centre of considerable public controversy in 2004 for getting a 'blow-dry' on a government trip to the US. 'We flew during the night on the government jet. We got in about 2 a.m. I was doing a media interview at 7 a.m.,' Harney recalls. An appointment was organised by others with a local hairdresser to come to the hotel to do Harney's hair ahead of the media interviews. The services that Harney received partially contributed to a $410 bill from the beauty salon. 'My God, it was really annoying. I mean, it was like as if I was trying to rip off the taxpayer,' she says.

For most female politicians, their appearance and dress code are simply part of the job. Gemma Hussey says she would 'worry like hell' about her appearance when she was Minister for Education as she was conscious of looking 'half-respectable' in front of the ever-present cameras. Despite the increased number of media outlets and more television coverage of politics in recent years, Hussey believes there was actually greater focus on the appearance of female politicians in the 1970s and 1980s as there were so few women in political life: 'Because I was the only woman around the cabinet table, they [the media] didn't have anybody to compare me with really. So in a way that was an advantage.'

Mary O'Rourke emerged into frontline political prominence in the same era as Hussey and was appointed Minister for Education in 1987: 'Of course, you would think of what you put on and what would be suitable.' She adds, 'I was conscious of my appearance. What woman isn't?' Charles Haughey, who appointed O'Rourke to cabinet, would often ask had she been 'shopping lately' to buy 'nice frocks'. O'Rourke never took offence: 'I thought he was trying to be nice [by] making a nice comment.'

Fine Gael's Nora Owen agrees with many of her colleagues that too much attention is given to appearance, although she recognises it is not something to neglect. Owen, who was Minister for Justice from 1994 to 1997, says, 'It's important you look smart, that you make an effort.' On days where she was 'under a lot of strain and looked a bit ragged, I would try to make time to slip out to have the hair done'. Hussey adopted a similar approach and luckily her hairdressers were located close to Leinster House: 'I would ring up and I would say, listen, if I was over in five minutes, can you do something?' O'Rourke says she was 'very lucky in that I have a head of hair, which I still have. So I was able to manage that myself always. I might go for a wash and blow-dry or whatever.'

As far as Owen is concerned, as a female politician her hair, make-up and clothes were part and parcel of her job. She had to adapt very quickly to this when John Bruton appointed her Minister for Justice in 1994. The Rainbow Coalition was formed without a general election being called: 'I became a minister overnight. I had a friend in the clothes business. I rang [the friend] and by the time I got home that night there was a number of outfits waiting for me.' In terms of her appearance, the new minister was very conscious of not letting herself down. Owen recalls her first official engagement and feeling one item of clothing missing: 'I didn't have gloves. And when I saw the picture – my two white hands are sticking out at the end of my coat. And I thought "Nora, you need gloves." And [afterwards] I never moved without a pair of gloves in the car.' Owen says she was very aware of her appearance as a government minister. 'Particularly with the gardaí, because the senior gardaí were always in gloves and hats – full uniform and all their gold and everything.'

The lesson learned about the value of gloves resurfaced more than a decade after Owen had left Leinster House. She was watching television coverage on the appointment of new ministers to the Fine Gael–Labour coalition in 2014 when news broke that Heather Humphreys, a first-time Fine Gael TD from 2011, was being appointed in the cabinet reshuffle. Shortly afterwards Owen rang the new minister: 'I knew she was going to be laying wreaths and everything. I said, "Heather, I'm going to give you a bit of advice" – because [at] her first function she was in a black suit, but she didn't have gloves on – "buy yourself a nice pair of black leather gloves and keep them in the glove compartment" [of the car].'

Humphreys laughs when reminded of the conversation. She says, 'that was good advice' about gloves finishing her outfit: 'I remember going into [Arnotts in Dublin] and the sale was on, and I bought myself the most beautiful pair of long black gloves. And I used to wear those when I was laying wreaths. And she [Owen] was dead right. Wear the gloves. And it looks better.'

While Frances Fitzgerald cannot recall what she wore the day she was first appointed to cabinet in 2011, she never discounted the importance of appearance when she was a minister. 'I always took the view that I wanted to look professional and be professional,' the Fine Gael politician says. Part of looking professional involved 'getting your hair done' and 'putting on make-up', but time was also a consideration: 'When you are as busy as I was, then you want to wear something that's easy every day. I would tend to wear jackets and a black dress or a navy dress because you really didn't have time to do very much shopping [so] you want something that you know works.' Mary Harney followed a similar approach with a preference for trouser suits: 'I find them more comfortable. It's the norm now. I mean, Angela Merkel nearly always wears trousers.'

Other female ministers adopted a more deliberate and political strategy especially for big personal occasions. On her first day as a TD, and later when she was appointed to cabinet, Mary Hanafin made sure that she ticked three boxes: 'female designer; local; green.' On both of those big days, Hanafin, whose family comes from Co. Tipperary, wore green outfits by the designer Louise Kennedy 'because she was [from] Thurles'. 'I nearly always wore green because it's kind of my republican leanings coming out,' she says.

Hanafin is not the only female politician who was conscious of selecting an outfit for their first day as a TD. Labour's Jan O'Sullivan remembers wearing 'a kind of periwinkle-coloured trouser suit, that kind of mauvey, purpley colour, nice and bright'. O'Sullivan says she chose the suit carefully: 'I did quite deliberately choose it because I knew this was a big moment and I wanted to look as well as I could.' She admits to having spent more on the outfit that would be her norm. Mary Coughlan also recalls the grey and black suit that she bought for her first day in the Dáil as it cost 'ten fortunes at the time'.

Fine Gael's Josepha Madigan did not have a lot of time to plan her outfit when she was appointed to cabinet in November 2017. Madigan had just dropped her children to school when Taoiseach Leo Varadkar relayed the news of her elevation from the Fine Gael backbenches to the cabinet table: 'I went straight out to Dundrum, bought an outfit and got my hair blow-dried.' 'Typical female,' she says, but adds, 'I knew I was going to be in photographs.' Madigan candidly admits the focus on appearance is 'a pain', but, like the other women who have been appointed as government ministers, accepts that it is also part of the job: 'I don't identify myself with how I look but society doesn't thank you for not looking well. I think it's part of being professional. You know, I think it can be difficult for women in terms of clothes and being appropriately dressed and not over the top. It's difficult.' Politics aside, Madigan says, 'I probably wouldn't be low cleavage and short skirt. I might have been twenty years ago but there's a balance, you know. And you don't want to be known for the wrong reasons. So I do think you need to be professional in how you dress.'

❧ ❧ ❧

The two women who have been elected president of Ireland were among the most photographed people in the country during their terms in office. For both Mary Robinson and Mary McAleese, it would have been impossible not to be conscious of their appearance.

At the very outset of her career in political life, Robinson was given advice on what to wear, advice that she now regrets taking: 'I came to the Senate wearing this ridiculous beret,' she recalls. Robinson was first elected to the Seanad in 1969. Her decision to wear a hat on her first day in the chamber had been influenced by a colleague who she met as she was going to sign the register: 'I met Senator Kit Ahern of Fianna Fáil. And she welcomed me, and she said, "Now don't forget, Mary, when we meet, which was in a few days' time, you have to wear a hat." And I completely believed her.' Robinson later found out this stipulation was not actually true: 'I discovered that it was ridiculous. I was so furious because, of course, every photograph of what I was doing or saying at that time had me in this beret.' She adds, laughing, 'I don't think I ever wore it again.'

Almost twenty years later, when Robinson set off on her presidential campaign trail in 1990, she was again the recipient of advice about her appearance. She was bluntly told that she 'needed a makeover'. At one event, one woman asked her 'if [she] had the wardrobe for [the job].' Robinson admits, 'I thought she meant a physical wardrobe.' As a presidential candidate, she was aware of her appearance and the advice was heeded. 'Image was important on the campaign trail. It's part of the job,' she says, adding, 'What I wanted was to get good advice, take it, deal with that issue and be done with it.' Robinson was also conscious of who designed her clothes: 'As president, I wore nothing but Irish clothes.' She also opted for high-neck jumpers and pearls but decided to abandon wearing trousers: 'As president, I didn't wear trousers except privately, you know, on holidays.' Since leaving Áras an Uachtaráin, that practice has ended and she has resumed wearing trousers.

As the first Irish woman elected president, Robinson's appearance attracted a lot of attention and not just at home. 'I was on the best-dressed list in the world for a while, would you believe?' she says. However, there were occasions when her dress code was not positively received. For example, she remembers attending the Melbourne Cup in Australia: 'I wasn't wearing a hat, I was wearing a very smart suit of course.' Her outfit stood out when she met the ladies' committee and 'every single one of them had large hats. And they looked at me in shock horror, that I wasn't wearing a hat. It was terribly funny, you know.'

While the reaction to her outfit on that occasion was unintended, Robinson sometimes used her appearance to make a very clear statement, as she did during a visit to the Vatican on International Women's Day. It is practice for Catholic women to wear black dresses and mantillas in the presence of the pope. Robinson, however, decided not to wear black, nor did she wear a veil. Instead, she opted for a dark green suit with a sprig of yellow mimosa, the symbol of International Women's Day. She recalls that there was 'a bit of a shock' at her choice among some of the Vatican officials. Pope John Paul II, she says, 'didn't mind at all'. A few months later, she visited him in her new role as UN High Commissioner for Human Rights wearing the same green outfit: 'He said, "I think you are wearing the same coat" and we laughed.' Both had clearly been conscious of the significance of her outfit on the previous visit.

Like Robinson, McAleese adopted a very pragmatic approach to her appearance: 'We are representatives at a very high level. It's an opportunity to showcase the best of Irish design and good Irish hairdressing and good Irish make-up, all of that. I had to subscribe to that. And I did. It was part of the job.' The idea of people commenting on what she wore was something she grew to accept, if not necessarily like. 'You have got to put up with all that nonsense,' she says, adding, 'You just have to take it.'

While in Áras an Uachtaráin, McAleese adopted a hands-off approach, placing complete trust in her team to choose her clothes: 'They were the oracles on that. I just let them tell me, "You are wearing this, you are wearing that." And that was it.' It will surprise many that this approach and level of delegation also extended to trips overseas: 'I got to the far end and I never knew what was in the suitcases.' Since leaving office in 2011, she says she can now 'relax a bit and tootle around in the jeans'. However, she admits there were some practical advantages to being president. During her two terms in the Áras, she never carried a purse or a mobile phone: 'I'm actually not a handbaggy person. I hate the darn things.'

❧ ❧ ❧

While the two presidents were very aware of showcasing the work of Irish designers, several female ministers openly accept they themselves can also benefit from the media and public focus on appearance.

At the local elections in 1985, Mary Hanafin was the only female Fianna Fáil candidate in her electoral area. She chose her clothes to stand out. Thirty years later, she remembers a conversation with Liz Allman, the wife of Labour's Ruairi Quinn: '[Liz] was slagging me, she said, "I remember you wearing a bright yellow suit"'. Hanafin stresses the advantage in being different from 'a sea of grey'. She believes it is a positive and that female candidates now 'play to it'. The former Fianna Fáil minister also believes there was a better chance of being on a television or radio programme because the producers wanted to have a gender balance. But the advantage comes with a caveat: 'I think you had to be more conscious of what you said and the way you said it, and how you looked while you were saying it.'

Like Hanafin, Labour's Niamh Bhreathnach saw some advantages in being a female minister: 'You were the only woman in a crowded room so there was an advantage about having a red coat on you.' It certainly got people's attention, she remembers: 'I once heard somebody saying that I was glamorous. And I turned around to see who was saying it. It was two nuns. I normally think glamorous people are thin and tall. It was quite funny.'

Being what Nora Owen calls 'a rare species' also had benefits: 'When you went somewhere, you were nearly always recognised, whereas lots and lots of male backbenchers could turn up and nobody would know the hell who they were.' Like some of the other female ministers, Owen took advantage of bright colours to stand out. Mary Coughlan also subscribed to this policy: 'If you were wearing pink and everybody else is wearing black, it wasn't hard to work out who was going to be seen.'

In a Dáil chamber that, even after the first gender-quota election in 2016, is still dominated by men, Regina Doherty is aware of the argument about wearing bright colours to stand out. 'I would have hated that,' she says. 'I don't wear bright pink or red. They wouldn't have been natural colours in my wardrobe at the time. But you very quickly find out that unless you stand out either by having a big mouth or being assertive, then you have to find other ways to stand out.'

The Fine Gael politician accepts there are 'swings and roundabouts' to the arguments about appearance. She often meets women in her constituency who comment on her outfits: 'They say, "Jesus, Regina, I was watching you on the television in that gorgeous pink jacket."' Doherty believes it is human nature to focus on somebody's appearance: 'I do it myself. If I'm watching the two women on the television, I'll go, "Oh Jesus, look at that lovely black frock she's wearing."' She admits she never particularly notices what a man is wearing: 'I couldn't give a hoot.'

❧ ❧ ❧

If female politicians get more attention as a result of their appearance, they also come under greater scrutiny. Most of the female ministers are of the firm view that 'double standards' are applied both by the public and the media when it comes to judging the appearance of politicians – and that men get off easier. Independent TD Katherine Zappone jokes that when it comes to dressing for the job, it's the only time she has flirted with the idea she would rather have been a man. 'Honest to God, it takes a lot of time and effort,' she says. 'I think that wouldn't be as positive if a woman didn't quite look up to par but the men get away with that …' But she is quick to point out that her male cabinet colleagues are 'spiffy dressers' before asking, 'aren't they?'

Mary Harney believes there are expectations placed on women that are not applied to men: 'You rarely see commentary about men. I know Bertie's anorak was the subject of commentary but it was the exception, [as was] Leo in his gym wear.' Generally, Harney says the excessive focus on appearance 'doesn't apply to men, it applies very much to women'. In her ministerial career from 1997 to 2011, Harney received considerable media attention: 'I saw commentary saying, Mary Harney wore this to this event and she wore that to this other event. Well, I wasn't going to go out buying something new for every event I went to.' She wonders 'would anyone notice if a man wore the same suit? No, definitely not.'

The media certainly noticed when this happened to former Tánaiste Frances Fitzgerald: 'I wore the same outfit twice [and] it was a headline in one of the newspapers.' Fitzgerald had gone to two events, one day after another: 'It's probably one of the few times I wore the same thing.' She was taken aback by the coverage: it was 'extraordinary that it was a story,' she says.

She doubts that her male counterparts would have come under such scrutiny. Mary Hanafin does not think male cabinet members would have received the same treatment as her either: 'The back of one of my dresses appeared on the front page of a tabloid,' she says, adding that it was part of a 'guess who is wearing this dress' competition. On seeing the photograph, her mother instantly said, 'That's Mary.' On another occasion, her shoes featured in a newspaper. 'They were great shoes, mind you,' she says, but adds: 'No man is going to get that.' And that was the point behind a tactic adopted by Mary Robinson's special advisor Bride Rosney, who was accustomed to dealing with media requests about the president's outfits in advance of state visits or trips. Robinson says Rosney often batted back such requests: 'Well if you tell me what the male incoming president will be wearing, who made his suit or that, I will let you know.'

Gemma Hussey shares this view that male politicians get off lightly in terms of preparation and scrutiny: 'I mean, you make a huge effort to always look neat, to have your face done and your hair done. [But] you would be conscious of all those men sitting around the [cabinet] table who weren't doing that ...' According to Nora Owen, the explanation is, in part, attributable to the fact that men 'wear a suit and a tie and shirt, or now they wear an open neck t-shirt that's bright pink or something and nobody seems to care'.

Máire Geoghegan-Quinn experienced these double standards from the very outset of her political career. When she won a by-election in Galway West in 1975, her Fianna Fáil colleague Michael Kitt was elected in a by-election in the neighbouring Galway North-East constituency. Shortly afterwards both new TDs entered the Dáil on the same day. 'There was that type of coverage [about] what I wore going into the Dáil but there was no talk about what Michael Kitt wore,' Geoghegan-Quinn recalls. Her 'signature look' at the time included 'boots up to my knees'. Coupled with her long hair, she remembers the knee-high boots attracting much attention. Geoghegan-Quinn recalls one female journalist who was fixated on her appearance and went on 'a one-woman rant' about her hair: 'She basically said that I was too old now to have my hair down long, because it was long and straight.' The journalist advised her to get it cut and styled. A friend of Geoghegan-Quinn's who grew tired of the commentary went as far as writing a letter of complaint to the journalist.

Some years later, Geoghegan-Quinn decided it was time to change her hairstyle: 'In the middle of the 1987 election campaign, I went to get my hair washed and I said to Maureen, who was doing my hair, I said "Do you know what, Maureen, I'm going to cut it up to the shoulder."' Her local hairdresser was 'very reluctant to do it because it was so long'. But Geoghegan-Quinn was determined that she 'get the scissors out' and 'cut it off'. On the campaign trail in Galway West, the reaction was immediate: 'The whole election became about Máire's hair. Did you see Máire's hair? Has anyone seen Máire's hair? It was in the paper. It was on the doorsteps – "Oh God, your hair is fabulous."' So, she says, 'it went back to the same thing all over again – appearance.' There was even a domestic response. 'I didn't even tell my husband [about getting it cut]. I came home and he was livid,' she laughs.

Aside from Bertie Ahern's anorak, Leo Varadkar's gymgear and Mick Wallace's pink shirts, there have been few exceptions to gendered commentary on appearance. The only man Geoghegan-Quinn remembers getting as much coverage on such matters was Ruairi Quinn. And that was due to 'his colourful ties', she says. The outcome is that female politicians end up having to be more careful about how they look in public. 'Men have a very standard way of dressing and that's [a] suit and tie. That's the norm for men,' says Heather Humphreys. 'I think women have to be careful that they don't trivialise their position by wearing things that are not appropriate.'

When Humphreys was elevated to cabinet in a reshuffle in 2014, she went out and bought some clothes specifically for her new role – no different than many women who get a promotion. However, Humphreys continued with the same dress code she had adopted in her previous professional life. She prefers 'to dress in a business-like manner because I'm doing a job. If I'm going to a party, I can dress up and wear fancy gear, if I so wish. But if I'm doing a job, if I'm to be taken seriously, I wear my suit or I wear a jacket and a dress. I wear what I consider to be professional.' The Cavan–Monaghan TD has a preference for dark colours, which has brought its own attention. On one occasion in her constituency, another woman remarked that 'she's never out of black'. Humphreys replied that if she had wanted to be a 'clothes horse', she would have chosen a different career.

The focus on clothes is heightened when female politicians are on television. Hanafin recalls getting feedback on 'whatever colour suit I had on that day' with comments such as 'love the colour', 'love seeing you in the chamber', 'the colour stands out.' There was also feedback on her make-up and hairstyle: '"Do you know your eye-shadow was the same colour as your lipstick?" And I would say, "Well, actually that's the RTÉ make-up department."' On another occasion, a woman went into a hairdresser in Hanafin's Dún Laoghaire constituency with a photograph of the Fianna Fáil minister and said: 'I want my hair cut the same as Mary Hanafin.'

Niamh Bhreathnach – who had represented the same constituency in the 1990s – had similar experiences. Outside of policy issues, Bhreathnach was asked most about her hair and, specifically, where she got it done. But not everyone is complimentary, as Jan O'Sullivan explains: 'People would say to me, "You should have got your hair done before you went on television."' Sometimes others would comment that 'you look better in real life than on television'. There would be far fewer comments on what she might have said during the television appearance. O'Sullivan says such comments were not just confined to members of the public and concedes that 'even male colleagues would talk about how you looked on television rather than what you said sometimes'. She adds, 'I don't think that happens to men. It probably happens to men like Mick Wallace.'

Mary Coughlan was a TD when regular televised coverage of Dáil proceedings started in the early 1990s: 'We were all briefed about what was appropriate to wear. I remember somebody saying don't wear dangly earrings, don't be wearing anything too low-cut.' Coughlan found the most significant changes to her dress code came about as her political role changed. In particular, there were new requirements when she was appointed Minister for Enterprise, Trade and Employment in 2008: 'One of the things that drove me scatty was when I was told in no uncertain terms that I could only wear black or grey.' She now accepts this was good advice: 'When you are meeting men and they want to take you seriously, you don't dress as flamboyantly.' Following a cabinet reshuffle in 2010, Coughlan moved to the Department of Education. 'Minister, you are expected to dress well but you can be as flamboyant and colourful as you want,' one senior civil servant advised.

Appearance aside, Coughlan found herself the focus of considerable media commentary when the economic crisis hit in 2008. The three senior government figures – Brian Cowen as Taoiseach, Brian Lenihan as Minister for Finance and Coughlan as Tánaiste – were under huge pressure to deal with the rapidly collapsing Irish economy: 'Brian Cowen would go out and do something. They [the media] would run around then to see what Brian Lenihan was going to say. And then they would run around town and see what I was going to say. The fact that I mightn't have spoken to Brian Lenihan or Brian Cowen about something happening in Finance – that didn't really impact on me. I would be asked, I wouldn't know the answer because I hadn't had bloody time to talk to Brian Lenihan because he hadn't time to talk to me. The herd was desperate. Everywhere I went, it didn't matter if I was going to the bathroom, you would have this influx of people running after you. They did the same to the two Brians. It was just desperate.' The moniker 'Calamity Coughlan' started to appear in newspaper headlines: 'It was easy and it stuck. And no matter what I did, if our Lord came off the cross, I was [not] going to change that. So I had to just take it and try to move on.' One response to the sustained negative media coverage was a total ban on newspapers in Coughlan's house.

Ironically, when it came to commentary on their appearance, there is a consensus among many of the women who have served as government ministers that female journalists tended to be their harshest critics. Nora Owen recalls 'some articles that would have said, she's not a great dresser or she hasn't a great sense of clothes.' She says they would describe set-piece days like the start of a new Dáil term: 'They would do a piece saying well, so-and-so had a rather nice lilac suit on and red seemed to be a favourite colour, and they would actually describe and pick out one or two outfits.' But, Owen adds, 'That's not really what parliament should be about. It shouldn't matter whether somebody had a rather nice lilac suit on or not. It's the fact that you are an elected member, exactly the same as the man sitting beside you, who is in the same suit for the last three days.' In terms of the 'social kind of stuff', Mary Harney agrees that 'some of the hardest people on me over the years would be women [in the] media'. She stresses she is referring to those writing 'the social kind of stuff'.

'I think the media reports women differently to the way they report men,' Frances Fitzgerald says. 'Assumptions are made about men in power that are not made about women in power. It's a different experience. It's a gendered experience, make no mistake about it.' During the 2016 general election campaign, Labour's Joan Burton experienced this type of media coverage after one of the televised leader debates. The former Labour leader recalls one commentator 'did not like the colour of my tights. They liked the outfit but they couldn't understand why I was wearing nude shiny tights.' Burton, however, took greater exception to a panel discussion on RTÉ television: 'I think it was a psychologist that *The Late Late Show* employed.' She says, 'Apparently whatever I did with my lips was an indication that I hadn't been breast-fed or something like that. It was completely weird.' She's not sure many men would have received such commentary: 'But given my own particular background [Burton is adopted], I thought it was pretty insensitive.' During her time as a government minister and party leader, Burton also found herself subject matter for political comedy programmes, although she considers this attention less invidious than commentary on her appearance: 'All the professional politicians will say to you, it is only when you become somebody who features in cartoons and features on Mario Rosenstock that you have achieved a certain status.' Her advice: 'Try and laugh at it when it's funny and just bite your lip when it's not.'

Overall, Burton accepts there is 'an awful lot of focus' on appearance but admits, 'to be honest, if people don't care for you, no matter what you do, even if you have a facelift, they still won't be impressed'. She sees the excessive prioritisation on the appearance of female ministers as a by-product of celebrity culture associated with glamour models: 'We are used to seeing incredibly beautiful women all done up. And expectations filter out to young girls and in respect to women politicians that actually you should look like this as well. And that's unlikely to happen.'

Mary Mitchell O'Connor's tenure as a senior cabinet minister from May 2016 to June 2017 was marked by a lot of media commentary and some criticism. One article even referred to her nails. 'I remember reading that article. We were coming back from a trade mission, and I was with the chief executive of the IDA. We had had a fantastic trade mission where there were promises of jobs,' she says. 'You need to ask the question of the person that would comment on my nails rather than me […] I was a minister in government. I did the job that Enda Kenny asked me to do.' Her Fine Gael colleague Regina Doherty firmly believes the coverage was sexist: 'So what if her nails are pink with diamonds on them? Who cares?'

Perceptions about appearance and reactions to the dress code of female politicians have changed significantly over the last forty years. For example, Nora Owen clearly remembers the day her Fine Gael colleague Avril Doyle wore leather trousers in Leinster House: 'The place nearly exploded. You could hear the intakes of breath as she came down the stairs [into the Dáil chamber] in the leather trousers.' Owen says that 'it caused quite a stir'. But she recalls the woman at the centre of this 'frisson' was not bothered: 'Oh, Avril to the manor born didn't mind.' Despite the audible reaction, Owen does not remember hearing any comments on Doyle's trousers: 'To be honest, the first time I ever heard that kind of comment in the chamber was from Mick Wallace [about] Mary Mitchell O'Connor.' Owen is referring to comments made by the Wexford TD Mick Wallace in 2011. During a private conversation with some colleagues in the chamber, Wallace referred to Mitchell O'Connor as 'Miss Piggy'. His remarks were caught on microphone, which caused some furore. Wallace promptly apologised to the Fine Gael TD. His apology was accepted and in the aftermath of the controversy, Mitchell O'Connor organised a charity photo-call to mark an end to what she described at the time as the 'rumble' in the Dáil. Mitchell O'Connor managed to turn the incident around. Seven years later, however, she admits the remarks were hurtful: 'Would you like it said about you?' Nora Owen sees a degree of unfairness at work: 'Have you ever heard the Taoiseach standing up and saying when Mick Wallace is making one of his big points, "I would take more heed of you if you dressed a bit better"?'

When the media were not commenting on how they looked, many female ministers also faced remarks from members of the public. Owen recalls going into Leinster House at summertime when she met a group of visitors: 'It was the middle of the summer and I normally would have had a jacket on if it was Dáil time.' She remembers the encounter clearly: 'I was wearing just a skirt and a blouse. And I was a lot slimmer then as well. I said hello to them and went on.' As she walked off, one woman in the group was overheard remarking on the appropriateness of Owen's attire: 'My God, wouldn't you think she would dress better.' The former Minister for Justice acknowledges how times have changed: 'Now, anything goes. I see Katherine Zappone in sleeveless dresses sitting in the chamber. Now I would never have done that in the 1980s or the 1990s. I would always have had a jacket on.'

7

FAMILY AND FRIENDS – CONSTANT GUILT

*I had two bags, one for going to Dublin and one that
I would pretend that I was staying. I would leave my
bag on my bed and my son Cathal would look at it and
think that Mammy was staying, and I would go out
the window and throw my bag in with the driver.*

MARY COUGHLAN

For TDs like Fianna Fáil's Mary Coughlan who represented a constituency outside Dublin, political life can be difficult. She spent part of the week in the capital away from her husband and children, who were living in Co. Donegal. For those who are considering entering politics, the impact on family life can be a deterrent.

Coughlan, though, knew the score. She had grown up in a political household – both her father and uncle had served as Fianna Fáil TDs. But, as a young mother with a young family, she describes leaving her family every week as 'horrible'. Ironically, Coughlan met her late husband, David Charlton, in Leinster House, where he was working as a garda. The couple set up home in Donegal and had two 'election babies', as the former Fianna Fáil minister calls them. Her son, Cathal, was born on the evening of the general election count in 1997. She vividly remembers the day: 'We were having a cup of tea and a sandwich afterwards, and I said to David, "I think I better move," and Cathal was born that night.' Two years later, her daughter, Maeve, arrived in the middle of the local elections in 1999, which Coughlan was contesting. 'She was born on Wednesday, I went home on Friday. David and my wee fella went down to stay with his mother for two weeks. And a young girl who turned out to be my nanny looked after Maeve until the election was over. I used to go and see her when I could. It was a mental way of going.'

The prospect of bringing her young children from Donegal to Dublin when the Dáil sat during weekdays was not feasible. She says that 'moving a child is like moving a house'. She had 'back-up at home' and her mother was a huge support: 'I was a minister and it was very difficult. And then my mother said, being the tough woman that she was, she says, "Mary, you have to know that when you go to Dublin, you can do nothing about what happens in Donegal. So whoever is in charge needs to be good." And I was very lucky. I had David, I had great nannies, and I had my mother and my sister.'

For most of the female ministers, trying to balance a political career and family life was difficult. There was the ongoing challenge of ensuring 'family time' was put into the ministerial diary, which was not always easy. 'You had to try and make sure with your secretary at the time that you got that hour or got home to do something. I remember driving down to Frosses, where I come from, which is a little village, and going to the nativity play and then going straight back up to Dublin. But I was there for the play. I would have been wrecked for two days after it, but I still would try and get to those things,' recalls

Coughlan. The round-journey of over 460 kilometres took almost seven hours.

With a busy constituency in Donegal South-West, Coughlan's political activities did not cease when she left Dublin. Her husband ensured that constituency callers went to her local office rather than coming to their home. But even when she was out locally with her children at weekends, there would be interruptions. She says her young children found this hard: 'They didn't like [that] you couldn't go anywhere when somebody would be talking to Mammy and you would be two hours waiting. You couldn't go to the shop.' There were still constituency calls even after she left national politics in 2011. But when the phone rang her daughter would remind her, 'Mammy, you are not in politics anymore.'

Looking back now, Coughlan is unsure how the Dáil can be reformed to make life for politicians more family-friendly: 'It's a bit nonsensical speaking about better working hours in the Dáil because that doesn't suit the country people. The country people like to kill themselves for three days in Dublin [and then go home].' With a family background in politics – and as someone who grew up in a political household – Coughlan sees politics as 'a way of life. And it doesn't fit into any other way of life. Trying to pigeonhole it into your way of life doesn't work.'

Most TDs from outside Dublin know the road from home to Leinster House and back again incredibly well. Fianna Fáil's Mary O'Rourke recalls the drive from her home in Athlone to Leinster House with a mantra: 'There was Moate and Horseleap and Kilbeggan and Tyrrellspass and Rochefort Bridge and Milltown Pass and Kinnegad and Enfield and Leixlip and Lucan and Dublin.' In the 1980s and 1990s, the absence of a motorway meant these car journeys were difficult. 'All those villages were becoming gradually clogged up, you know. They were long journeys. Now you get into your car and zoom, you are up on the highway,' she says.

In the early part of her political career, O'Rourke, who was the mother of two children, would frequently commute daily between Athlone and Dublin. But eventually, having discussed the travelling with her late husband, Enda, she decided to stay in Dublin mid-week: 'Enda said, "I think you will be found dead on the road if you keep coming home at 8.30 p.m. and 9 p.m. at night. What's the point? You don't see the children."' O'Rourke duly booked into Buswells Hotel when she was in Leinster House.

Máire Geoghegan-Quinn also remembers the impact on her young family. When she was first elected in 1975, she would drop off her son with her mother-in-law who lived in Tuam, before continuing on to Dublin: 'He would stay with her Tuesday night and Wednesday night and then on Thursday when I would be coming home, I would come via Tuam, and come back to Galway. We did that for probably a year, maybe a little bit more. And then we decided, why don't we get this babysitter to come, and she can live in Monday to Friday, and she will be there and she will look after him and take him to school, and all of that. Because my husband John worked the whole west coast from Clare all the way to Donegal. So, you know, if he was in Donegal, he wouldn't be coming home that night […] And when there was weekend stuff that I had to do, I would leave him with my mother, as she lived in the city as well.'

When her second child was born, Geoghegan-Quinn made further arrangements: she would 'take the baby with me on a Tuesday morning [to Dublin] and bring him home on a Thursday night. When I was in cabinet, sometimes we would go on a Monday evening and mightn't come home until Friday.' There were times when the first women to be appointed to cabinet since the foundation of the state questioned why she had not stayed as a teacher, asking herself, 'Oh God Almighty, what am I doing this for?' She contrasted her hours and lifestyle as a politician with her friends in her previous teaching job: '[We] were in at 9 a.m., finished at 2.30, no work to be done in the afternoon, only prep for the following day. We were off every Saturday and Sunday and we had long holidays and all the rest of it. And it's "Oh God, why did I get into this [political] job?"'

Guilt is an emotion many of the female ministers reference when they consider the impact their political careers had on home life, especially when they had young children. Geoghegan-Quinn admits to having felt 'constantly guilty'. She recalls one incident when her son Cormac, who was eighteen months at the time, had a small accident. Her husband had to bring him to hospital: 'When I came home I saw his little finger all bandaged and all the rest of it. And I said, "What happened to him?" My husband said, "Oh, he got his finger caught in something and we were in the hospital."' She immediately 'got into this whole guilt thing'. She says her husband, John tried to reassure her: 'It would have happened if you were here, like what are you getting upset about?' But she found that parking those emotions was easier said than done.

Niamh Bhreathnach recalls attending a Labour meeting when Dick Spring was party leader, before she was elected as a TD. It was Pancake Tuesday. She had woken up early that morning to prepare pancake batter before leaving for Leinster House. The meeting with Spring, due to start at 2 p.m., was put back to 4 p.m., by which time her children were due home from school and would have expected to be enjoying their pancakes: 'I had to take the decision. Dick Spring doesn't know it's Pancake Tuesday … [But] I knew if I got up and left the room to go home and make the pancakes, I would not be at the next meeting.' Her children were not impressed.

Gemma Hussey was the mother of three teenagers when she was appointed Minister for Education in late 1982. She knows she was fortunate in being a Dublin TD but still anticipated the challenges involved. The family sat down together to consider the implications of this elevation. 'I'm not going to be here. I'm going to be a missing entity for years,' Hussey told them frankly. She says her children were delighted and adds that they probably thought 'freedom at last'. She is equally grateful for the support of her husband, Derry, in facilitating her ministerial career: 'He's a traditional man from a traditional background. It was remarkably generous of him that it never bothered him. I mean he was encouraging from day one.'

She is not alone in terms of the support that she received – all the women who attained senior office proudly acknowledge the encouragement of their families in helping them to fulfil their political ambitious. Regina Doherty arrived at the cabinet table three decades after Hussey. The Fine Gael TD for Meath East has four children, the youngest of whom was four years old when she was first elected to the Dáil in 2011. She acknowledges her domestic support network and the role of her husband, Declan. She says if he was the type of husband who wanted his dinner on the table at 6 p.m. every evening, the couple 'would be divorced or he would have another wife'. She recognises the additional challenge for TDs living further from Dublin and mentions the case of Áine Collins, a Fine Gael TD for Cork North-West from 2011 to 2016: 'I would have been very close to Áine Collins when she was here. And Áine used to leave her babies on a Tuesday morning and not see them until a Friday morning because by the time she would get home on a Thursday evening, they would be gone to bed. Like her kids were as small as mine, when we were here for the first five years. And I'm not sure I could do that.'

The decision to move Dáil voting from Wednesday night to daytime on Thursdays improved family life according to Doherty, who was Government Chief Whip when the change was introduced: 'I would get home on a Wednesday night. We would vote here [in the Dáil] at 9 p.m. I would be home by 9.45. And that would be the earliest night that I would get home during the week – that was mine and Declan's night,' Doherty recalls. But, she suggests, even these changes have not totally lessened the demands on her time.

When asked about the impact of her political career on family life, Mary Mitchell O'Connor replies, 'I would nearly say back to you, "What family?" because you are away from them so much. I had a grandchild in 2017, and I think I counted that I had seen her five times in the year.'

Many of the women who were appointed senior ministers are very open about the pressure they felt in meeting work and family commitments. Frances Fitzgerald says, 'I'm sure I nearly crashed the car many a time getting out to events.' She is frank about the challenges of trying to balance family life and a political career: 'You kill yourself getting out to first communion events and choirs and the parent–teacher meetings were always a nightmare.' Fitzgerald was a young mother with three children under ten years of age when she was elected to the Dáil in 1992. The Fine Gael politician admits her domestic situation was easier because she was a Dublin-based TD, but there were still challenges with three young children: 'You still need good supports. You need childcare. It's expensive. It's very demanding. I mean, one of the things nobody ever writes about in Ireland is the number of women who have come and gone in this parliament. When I think of the number of women who have come in here for one term, and who have left – very common.'

The former Fine Gael minister highlights a specific occasion when one of her sons hurt himself with a firework: 'It's the one time I did cry, actually. And my two kids, the other lad fainted when he went in with the other guy in A&E. The person who was looking after them had brought them to Temple Street Hospital.' When she was contacted about the incident, Fitzgerald told the Chief Whip she had to leave Leinster House: 'You can't. You can't leave,' he replied, as the voting situation was so tight in the Dáil and the government could not afford to lose a vote. 'I started crying. I was so shocked. I was just overcome, because I was so concerned about what was wrong with my son,' Fitzgerald recalls. In this period, it would have been a significant political event for a government to lose a Dáil vote. Fitzgerald was freed to leave Leinster House an hour later. She says her son was fine.

Reflecting on her political career, Fitzgerald says she was initially disappointed when John Bruton overlooked her for a junior ministerial appointment when the Rainbow Coalition was formed in late 1994. She was first appointed to cabinet in 2011 but now recognises the personal benefit of this wait: 'Looking back, I'm really pleased it came to me at a later point in my career. Because I worked, you know, fifteen, eighteen hours a day as Minister for Justice and in the other ministries. People work incredibly hard. I think it's close to impossible to combine the highest level of ministry with the kind of family life that I would want.'

By the time Jan O'Sullivan was elected as a Labour TD for Limerick East in 1998, her daughter was in college in Dublin and her son was in secondary school. O'Sullivan says the situation would have been even more challenging had her children still been in primary school. 'I actually don't believe I would have run for a national election when they were in primary school,' O'Sullivan admits.

Heather Humphreys has a similar view to O'Sullivan and Fitzgerald about arriving at the cabinet table when her children had reached their teenage years. 'I think that would have been a price too high for me, in terms of not being able to be with the girls, if they were smaller. I would have missed out,' Humphreys says. The real pressure points, she feels, are in the evenings and at weekends – when political meetings and constituency activities eat further into family time. But Humphreys believes the same pressures apply to her male colleagues. One male TD told her he had been able to attend his child's Christmas play this year, and 'the excitement the child had, because his daddy was there'. This is in contrast to Gemma Hussey's experience of life as a TD in the 1980s, when, she says, most of her male counterparts left home and children for Leinster House, and 'never gave it a second thought in those days'.

Mary Harney, whose career in national politics covered the period from 1977 to 2011, still believes politics is 'tougher for women, particularly women that don't live close to Dublin and have to stay over in hotels' while working in Leinster House: 'One of the things that women colleagues would say to me over the years was "I really hate being away from the kids so much." In all my years in Leinster House I don't think any man ever said that to me. So there's a certain guilt that people feel. I didn't have children obviously, so I wasn't in that space. [But] the lifestyle itself is not family-friendly.'

Joan Burton has witnessed changed attitudes since she first won a Dáil seat in 1992. In the past, she says, quite a few of her male counterparts admitted to her that they 'missed all their children's communions, confirmations and so on because of commitment to Dáil business', whereas today, she says, they attend these events: 'I mean it would take some incredible, important and significant state issue that would stop somebody now attending a significant family event.' Burton, who was a senior minister from 2011 to 2016, tried to keep from mid-afternoon on Saturday and as many Sundays as possible free for her immediate family. She acknowledges, however, that time with family is sacrificed by those in political life, and says most politicians are dependent on 'very understanding and supportive families and friends'. Burton also ensured she took holidays: 'I think that's really important. Nobody is going to thank you. And again, when I came into the Dáil there were large numbers of politicians who never took a holiday. Their holiday was the constituency.'

Within weeks of being appointed to cabinet at the end of 2017, Josepha Madigan experienced the time demands that consume all government ministers. The Dublin–Rathdown Fine Gael TD has two teenage sons and she says 'the hardest part is on your family. And I think that's the same for everyone.' She says she 'was going to actually get a hologram and put it in the kitchen to say you actually have a mother.' Like the other female cabinet members, she acknowledges the importance of support from family in facilitating the work of being in cabinet: 'You are trying to make a difference and there's a lot of attention around that. But you have the husband or wife at home, who is doing the rugby, Gaelic and soccer, and the lunches and all of that.' Madigan tries to make the big family events, but adds, 'I didn't make the recent parent–teacher meeting last week. I couldn't do it. So Finn [her husband] did it.' She tries to have some level of demarcation between work and home: 'I'm Mum when I go home,' adding, 'My husband is interested for me, but he's not really interested in politics. So we talk about family things, which is nice.'

Madigan is conscious though of the 'emotional labour', which the former US presidential candidate Hillary Clinton mentions in her memoir of the 2016 campaign. Clinton highlighted the questions female politicians have to consider, such as does my child have a birthday present for the party on Saturday? Is the meat taken out of the freezer? 'These are the little things', Madigan says 'that are unquantifiable, that a woman is going to have to think of when she comes home at 11 o'clock at night, that no matter how wonderful her partner or husband is, you know. And it's not to cast aspersions on them, but they don't think of those things.'

❧ ❧ ❧

A number of women who have served as ministers suffered the loss of a spouse while in office. The public nature of their roles added additional pressures at such a personal time. However, some recount the kindness of colleagues from across the political divide. Mary Hanafin was Government Chief Whip when her husband Eamon Leahy, senior counsel and advisor to Fianna Fáil, passed away. She had been travelling on government business when word of his death reached her in July 2003. When the plane landed she remembers the scene: 'I mean the whole cabinet was there when I got off the plane in Dublin airport.' She appreciated the support of her political colleagues over the following months. 'You don't often see that side of people,' she says. '[There were] a few people I could ring up and say, "Look, are you going to the bar for a cup of coffee?" and they would always be there. You could link in with them, which was nice.'

It was a hugely difficult time. On one occasion, Hanafin recalls leaving a meeting in Government Buildings after a comment by a colleague 'kind of upset me a bit'. A couple of hours later, she got a call from the Taoiseach Bertie Ahern. 'He rang me from the government jet. He said, "I saw you got a little bit upset there, are you alright?" And I just thought it was so nice.' Hanafin says she wasn't capable of doing any media interviews for over six months. When she did her first interview following her husband's death, she remembers afterwards leaving 'the studio in tears because suddenly your whole world comes crashing in on top of you'.

When Katherine Zappone's wife, Ann Louise Gilligan died in June 2017, she recalls similar empathy – what she describes as 'unbelievable kindness' – from her cabinet and Dáil colleagues: 'I really felt embraced – embraced is a strong word – but I did feel that way from most of them, from men as well as women. I suspect, you know, it is because I demonstrated my emotion and so that pulls that out of people.' Zappone and Gilligan married in Canada in 2003. They had both actively campaigned for same-sex marriage here and when it was clear that the marriage equality referendum in Ireland was going to be passed in 2015, Zappone proposed to Gilligan during a live television programme covering the referendum results. Less than a year later, Zappone won a Dáil seat and was appointed to cabinet. Following her bereavement, she was very open in demonstrating her emotions. 'Because I'm a woman, because I was so soft about it, I was very vulnerable. A lot of men don't demonstrate that kind of vulnerability as easily,' she says, adding that her political colleagues 'responded positively to that vulnerability, which is great.'

❀ ❀ ❀

'I was married to politics. It was my job. It was my social life. It was my family, if you like,' Mary Harney says. The former Progressive Democrats minister married Brian Geoghegan in 2001 but for most of her political career she was single: 'Any job that has you in the public domain at a higher level, as you go up the career ladder, whether lonely is the word or not, I think it's challenging. But it's probably more challenging for a woman, I think.'

Harney counts a period in the 1980s during the heaves against Fianna Fáil party leader Charles Haughey as 'the most unpleasant' period of her political career. It was also very difficult on her family. 'Very, very nasty things were said to undermine people,' she says. In particular, Harney recalls untruthful rumours invented about her sexual behaviour with a colleague: 'So was I happy with them? Definitely not. Was I devastated by them? No.' She says pragmatically, 'You just have to be tough, and very determined and not lose focus.' But, she adds, 'I have no doubt they were damaging,' adding 'I mean, you know this phrase, "there's no smoke without fire".' These types of rumours and innuendo she believes, while not gender specific, are 'more damaging to a woman than a man'.

Harney was elected leader of the Progressive Democrats in 1993: 'It was lonely. I mean, I was a single person then. Obviously, for the last seventeen years I'm in a different position. With a partner, it makes life, you know, so different.' As a party leader, she believes there are restrictions in terms of those colleagues who can be involved in confidential discussions: 'You have got to be very careful who you can confide in and all members of the parliamentary party have to be treated the same. So you can't go to one with your woes and get their advice. You have to lead everybody and be fair to everybody. So I would have relied a lot on Des [O'Malley] for advice'. And that is still the case. 'More recently when I was asked to become the Chancellor of the University of Limerick', she says, '[and] he was the one I sort of said to, "What do you think?" I just like his opinion. I mightn't always agree with it. I might actually do the opposite, but I would like to hear it.'

Part of the isolation and loneliness of political life is attributed by Nora Owen to the fact that politicians tend to be sole traders: 'We are part of a party but we are essentially sole traders. It is a lonely thing. And when you leave politics, you realise that there's really only three or four or five people that you actually could meet again. I mean, when I go into the Dáil, everybody says "hello" and I say "hello" to everybody. But I'm not ringing them up regularly, I'm not meeting them regularly.' The former Fine Gael Minister for Justice says there are only four or five former Dáil colleagues who she would view as friends. She says the life of a TD and minister is 'lonely enough and you seldom would be very friendly with the person in your own constituency, because the competition is so great'.

Mary Mitchell O'Connor also recognises this aspect of political relationships. 'You sink or swim. You know, everyone is an adult.' She adds, 'You have to deliver, you have to do the job, [but] it's a lonely life.' Many female ministers from an earlier era agree with this conclusion. Gemma Hussey admits to having been 'quite lonely' when she was a government minister, despite the political support network in her party and department: 'I didn't really have somebody to really confide in.' While Hussey had very good female friends in Leinster House with whom she remains friends with today, she says many of her close friends were not in politics. For her, there was a lack of 'people to talk to, soulmates. I certainly felt that.' As the only female Independent minister around the cabinet table in the Fine Gael–Independent minority government, Katherine Zappone says she 'feels lonely at times'. She counts many of her ministerial and Dáil colleagues as friends, but she is very conscious of her status as a 'non-aligned Independent minister' and 'the only Independent woman at the cabinet table'.

Irrespective of political allegiances, the situation is lonelier for many female TDs from rural constituencies than those representing Dublin constituencies, according to Mary Hanafin: 'If you are in Dublin, you are getting home every night. And that makes a big, big difference. If you are from the country you are in a hotel or you are in your flat. It's a completely different situation.'

Máire Geoghegan-Quinn, a TD for Galway West from 1975 to 1997, says she was lucky in her early years in that she stayed with close friends from outside the world of politics who were living in Dublin. She eventually ended up moving in with Ann Ormonde, who was a Fianna Fáil senator: 'I had been very good friends of her brother, when he was a TD. And then when Ann was elected to the Seanad, we became great friends and she said, "Look, you know, I have spare rooms in the house, why would you be going to a hotel when you can stay with me?"'

The importance of having friends outside politics is mentioned by many of the female ministers. In her early days in the Dáil, Fianna Fáil's Síle de Valera would get her non-political friends to meet her in Leinster House: 'Many of my friends ended up coming into the Dáil for a cup of tea because I couldn't go out, because of voting. Your time was very much restricted but then that goes with the job.' Jan O'Sullivan recognises that working in Leinster House can be lonely when you are away from home for days on end. She says she would tend to 'mix with a small number of people' in Leinster House but her approach is to 'work when I'm up here, and I do my socialising when I'm in my constituency with my own friends'.

While Heather Humphreys says 'I'm not lonely. I have colleagues that I'm friendly with', she shares the view that politicians irrespective of their political background 'are sole traders really. Because when you go up for election you are on your own, you are pitted against your party colleague or you are pitted against the opposition. When you are in this business here, you have to make your own decisions.' While acknowledging the support provided by political parties, she says, 'You are on your own.' Leinster House can be a tough place, according to Frances Fitzgerald: 'I haven't felt lonely but I think it's tough. It's very tough.'

❧ ❧ ❧

Dáil Éireann was particularly tough for women holding ministerial or front-bench positions in the 1980s, according to the women who served in cabinet during this era. Mary O'Rourke and Gemma Hussey were political sparring partners at the time. O'Rourke says she had a 'sister fellow feeling' towards her Fine Gael counterpart, who was a cabinet minister from 1982 to 1987 before leaving national political life in 1989. O'Rourke was first appointed to cabinet in 1987. The two women were born a year apart (O'Rourke in 1937; Hussey in 1938). Both were students at Loreto Convent in Bray. During their time as political rivals, they had an understanding – they sparred, but they didn't scream at each other. Hussey says they 'made a kind of an agreement that we weren't going to shriek and roar at each other. We were not going to let anybody talk about cat fights, and all that kind of stuff. We weren't going to do that. And so we didn't do it.' O'Rourke concurs: 'We never said it but I think we kind of felt it between us. It was hanging there, you know.'

Hussey moved portfolios in a botched cabinet reshuffle in 1986 with Garret FitzGerald switching the Wicklow politician – against her preference – from Education to Social Welfare. Ironically, O'Rourke, her political rival, sent her a note saying she was sorry to see what had happened. 'She was very confident, and very good as Minister for Education, I remember thinking, now that's an awful thing they have done to her,' O'Rourke recalls.

Hussey was the only woman at cabinet in FitzGerald's second coalition administration. She says she got on well with Austin Deasy, the Fine Gael Minister for Agriculture: 'We sat beside each other. And he was terribly funny. He would write me notes. Garret would have very long, convoluted meetings. I mean the meetings went on forever.' On one occasion, Deasy passed Hussey a piece of paper on which he had written: 'Do you know what they are talking about, Gemma, because I don't?' She laughs, recalling, 'We would throw our eyes up to heaven.'

Party-political differences have often derailed the prospect of a strong sisterhood developing in Leinster House. But Nora Owen speaks for many female ministers when she references 'a sort of a sisterhood'. Máire Geoghegan-Quinn highlights this as well, when she says there is 'a kind of a sisterhood' but not a very strong one. Mary Harney recalls, 'If you came into the members' bar in the latter years for a coffee, you might be more inclined to join a woman if she was there, just the way nature is, I suppose.' Niamh Bhreathnach remembers Harney inviting her to join her for tea, although she says 'philosophically we would be streets apart'.

Frances Fitzgerald suggests that links between female politicians are 'not any way as developed as they could be'. She firmly states that allegiances in Leinster House break down on party lines: 'Party always wins out.' She also believes that that 'political friendships are different to other friendships'. Do they last? 'I'm not sure about that,' is her first response, before she adds, 'some of them do'.

Over the years there have been occasional social events organised for female politicians, but ultimately party politics come to the fore. 'Finding an issue where we could all travel the same path was quite difficult,' Nora Owen admits. Katherine Zappone says she made some efforts to bring female politicians together when she was a senator, without any success: 'I didn't get anywhere.' As for a sisterhood existing in Leinster House, Zappone states, 'Well, I would like to be part of it if there is.'

Zappone welcomes the establishment of the new women's caucus, which brings the increased number of female Oireachtas members together. 'I think that's a good idea', Jan O'Sullivan says. 'It's cross-party and it's considered to be a safe space where you know women can get together and talk about the various things we want to achieve in here.' A test of its success will be the level of unity it maintains. If it weathers the dynamics of party politics and survives in years to come, it will ultimately be judged on its ability to affect further change from inside a system that is still male-dominated.

CONCLUSION – A
CHANGING IRELAND

To help the women obtain their freedom.

COUNTESS CONSTANCE MARKIEVICZ

O ver the last half-century, there have been seismic changes in social and political attitudes in Ireland. These important changes did not come about by accident, but followed years of campaigning and pressure in the streets as well as the legal and political systems. In many respects, Mary Robinson's election as head of state in 1990 marked a turning point for the role of women in Irish society. At that time, Ireland was still a country where divorce was banned and access to contraception was still restrictive. Twelve months after Robinson's election, the Virgin Megastore in Dublin was fined for selling condoms. In 1992, a High Court ruling prevented a fourteen-year-old rape victim with suicidal thoughts from travelling to England to have an abortion. A national debate tied up with the constitutional referendum in 1983 was reignited. The High Court ruling was overturned by the Supreme Court. The debate, however, on abortion continued, culminating in Irish voters casting their ballots in numerous referendums in 1992, 2002, and 2018, when the electorate emphatically decided to delete the Eighth Amendment from the constitution and give the Oireachtas the power to legislate on the issue.

Most of the female ministers who have sat at the cabinet table have lived through dramatic changes on issues such as abortion, contraception, divorce and homosexuality. The place of women in Irish life, as well as in the world of politics, has been transformed. While not in every way, and not always as fast, as many would like, it is difficult to argue that there has not been huge change. At nineteen, the number of women who have sat at the cabinet table in almost one hundred years is pitiful (September 2018). But the environment, both domestic and international, in which we are now discussing such matters has changed, with greater priority being placed on issues important to women, including female representation. To put it simply, the mood music has changed.

In the past, outside influences helped to trigger major shifts in policies and attitudes. The experience of these female politicians reinforces this point and provides perspective to the current debate on the promotion of women in politics. Over the last half-century, pressure from the courts, the influence of the European Union following Irish membership in 1973, the decreasing power of the Catholic Church along with a younger and better-educated population have influenced how the occupants of Leinster House and Government Buildings address issues around rights, equality and diversity in both political debates and policy-making.

❧ ❧ ❧

As a member of Seanad Éireann since the late 1970s, Fine Gael's Gemma Hussey introduced a private members' bill that attempted to widen the definition of rape in criminal law. Hussey recalls how controversial the subject matter was at the time. In response to her call for the definition to be radically extended, one senator remarked that many women 'upset the biological balance of a man and then claim they were raped'.[43] The language associated with sexual abuse, Hussey remembers, made many politicians very uncomfortable. At that time, the vast majority of senators were men. Hussey says many of her male colleagues 'were embarrassed' when she first raised the issue. 'I knew I was going to have to say words like vagina and penetration. And I was nervous about it,' she admits. To counter any hostility in the chamber, Hussey ensured she had lots of support in the public gallery of the Seanad: 'All the senators could see that the gallery was absolutely full of women. And they daren't say anything.'

There were also some uncomfortable moments at the cabinet table when Hussey served in government from 1982 to 1987. The depressed state of the Irish economy and continually poor public finances dominated many ministerial meetings of the Fine Gael–Labour coalition. Hussey, the lone woman at cabinet, recalls a 'kind of shuffling' among her male ministerial colleagues when she attempted to make the case to remove VAT from sanitary towels. It was 'a rather strange moment', she admits. Hussey maintains her admiration for Garret FitzGerald for the progressive attitudes he espoused and promoted as Fine Gael leader and Taoiseach, but she is very much of the view that her job would have been different if there had been more women at cabinet. 'I mean you wouldn't have been fighting a lone battle,' she says.

❖ ❖ ❖

Mary Robinson was an early leader of the political and social liberalisation and secularisation of Irish society that had been underway since the 1960s. When she was first elected to the Seanad in 1969, as an Independent member representing Trinity College, Robinson was one of a handful of female senators, out of a cohort of sixty. There were men who supported her plans to introduce legislation on women's rights and other equality issues, including Trevor West and John Horgan, but they were minority voices. 'We really had no influence on the agenda,' she admits. Robinson recalls proposing her first private members' bill in 1971, which addressed the ban on the sale of contraceptives: 'I had an early example of how incredibly against the culture, if you could put it that way, it was to table a bill to amend a criminal law bill on family planning.' Her bill faced significant obstruction in even being debated, not to mind being passed. 'It sat there and couldn't get a first reading. Usually the first reading is automatic,' she recalls.

Robinson made seven attempts in 1971 to have her bill read in the Seanad. It could not be printed and published without a first reading.[44] 'And then I was told one morning that it was going to be taken at lunchtime,' Robinson recalls. Her opponents intended to kill the family planning bill without providing adequate notice for a real debate. 'We were voted down. And we switched to calling it the health family planning bill, and added in some family health issues to the legalising of contraceptives and removal of the criminality of condoms,' Robinson says. Her persistence met 'with condemnation in the press and on the pulpit in particular, [and] there was also condemnation in the House.' Brendan Corish, who was Labour leader and 'a very nice man', offered Robinson some friendly advice: 'Mary, I don't think this legislation is a good idea. I would advise you not to put it forward.' She was also criticised by the local bishop in Co. Mayo. Her parents 'had to walk out of mass in Ballina.' Robinson decided to ask Cardinal William Conway, the Catholic primate of

All Ireland, to intervene and send a message of support for her mother and father. His response, she remembers, was 'very cold, very unsupportive'. He replied, 'I will pray for them.' Robinson doubts a male politician would have been treated in this way: 'There was the power of the church, and I was a woman.'

As historian J.J. Lee notes, public attitudes on the liberalisation of Ireland's laws on contraception began to shift in the 1970s and 1980s with 'contraception superseding celibacy.'[45] One study of social attitudes published in 1977 showed that while 57.6 per cent agreed that premarital sex was always wrong, 63 per cent disagreed that it was always wrong to use artificial contraceptives.[46] During these years, debates about social issues and women's role in society became more pronounced in the political sphere. But many female ministers recall that, as in wider Irish society, these debates took place in an atmosphere in Leinster House that was often hostile. Mary Harney was appointed to the Seanad in 1977 and won a Dáil seat as a Fianna Fáil candidate for the first time in 1981. As a young woman, she was uncomfortable with the conservative stance that her party adopted on key social issues such as the greater liberalisation of contraception legislation and removing the constitutional prohibition on divorce legislation. Harney was equally frustrated that the party whip was applied to Dáil votes on such matters: 'We had no divorce, we had no comprehensive family planning and we had the 1983 [abortion] amendment. All those things made me feel very uneasy. I was in a completely different space. I felt there were times when I shouldn't be there.' She recalls John Wilson, when he was a government minister, asking another Fianna Fáil colleague: 'That Mary Harney one is obsessed with contraception and divorce. What's wrong with her?'

Harney ultimately split with Fianna Fáil and, with her political mentor, Des O'Malley, founded the Progressive Democrats.

O'Malley's stance on liberalising the contraception laws led to his expulsion from Fianna Fáil. However, Harney notes O'Malley's initial social conservatism: 'I first started reading Des O'Malley's speeches when he was the Fianna Fáil spokesperson on health. He was talking about fornication and all kinds of things. Jesus, he was so conservative. [But] I think he met a lot of younger people with me – and his own family, his children – that changed his attitudes on some of those issues. He was a person that evolved in that space.' Reflecting on that period, Harney also takes issue with some of the media coverage and believes there was a bias: 'Men would be asked their opinions on the North or the economy. [The media] would focus on the women on divorce, contraception, abortion, anything to do with family.'

For women's groups, these social issues were a priority and they actively campaigned to change the legal ban on contraceptives. For some advocates and opponents, this battle may have been viewed as the first step in effecting change in other important areas. In May 1971, on World Communications Day, a trip to Belfast organised by the Irish Women's Liberation Movement to buy contraceptives in defiance of the laws at the time, became known as the Condom Train. It attracted considerable controversy. [47] But their actions demonstrated that those campaigning for change would not be quiet.

A decision of the Supreme Court in 1973 led to a change in Ireland's contraception laws. Mary McGee, a 27-year-old mother of four who had been advised that another pregnancy would put her life at risk, took a legal challenge after contraceptives ordered from abroad were seized by Customs. The Supreme Court ruled that McGee had a right to marital privacy under the Constitution. It would take another six years before politicians legislated to change the law, and even then, it was a restrictive proposal. The eventual political solution was the infamous 'Irish solution to an

Irish problem'. To give effect to the judgement, the Minister for Health, Charles Haughey, introduced legislation that essentially meant only married couples had access to contraception – a doctor's prescription was required and this could only be provided to those seeking contraception for bona fide family planning purposes.

Máire Geoghegan-Quinn recalls her frustration at later attempts to maintain the strict parameters of that legislation. In 1985, Labour Minister for Health Barry Desmond in effect proposed liberalising the legislation that Geoghegan-Quinn's party leader, Haughey, had introduced. Desmond proposed changing the law to allow condoms to be sold by certain designated outlets to anyone over eighteen years of age without a prescription. As Fianna Fáil leader in 1985, Haughey wanted his party to oppose Desmond's proposal. When the issue came to the Fianna Fáil parliamentary party, Geoghegan-Quinn was one of those who refused to support Haughey's stance. On the day of the meeting, the Galway West TD was ill. She recalls getting, 'out of my sick bed with laryngitis [and] whispering almost in the parliamentary party meeting. But I spoke at length.' She told her colleagues that opposing Desmond's plan was 'ridiculous'. Haughey's view, however, prevailed. After the meeting, he approached Geoghegan-Quinn. 'He tapped me on the shoulder, and he said, "Máire, I was very sorry for you this morning with that laryngitis". Geoghegan-Quinn was not impressed. 'I said, "No, all you are sorry for is that I ever turned up so that I could talk."' The legislation was passed by the Oireachtas in spite of Fianna Fáil's opposition.

When issues such as the contraception came before the Dáil, Nora Owen, who was on the Fine Gael backbenches for most of this era, characterises the debates that took place as 'very Catholic'. Despite political resistance, she remembers growing pressure from the public to liberalise the law. 'Women began to realise they didn't want to just keep having children,' Owen says. But even in her Dublin North constituency there were differing views. One woman, a mother of six children, was outspoken in her opposition when she visited Owen's weekly clinic. 'Oh, I don't really want that,' she told the Fine Gael TD. 'I would have to make decisions, and I would have to decide if it's God's will that he [her husband] wants to have sex when he comes home and I get pregnant. Well, it's God's will.'

Labour's Jan O'Sullivan faced similar views when commencing her political career in Limerick. She recalls the campaign for a family planning clinic in the city in the late 1970s. 'It was very much frowned upon by the vast majority of people,' she recalls, adding that the campaigners were seen as 'pariahs in society at the time'. 'There was fierce opposition,' she explains. 'The Catholic Church was such a dominant force at the time. It was considered to be interfering in family life and the kind of morals that people had been taught.' She remembers seeing people reciting prayers outside the clinic in protest.

Other female politicians experienced hostility, especially when the introduction of the Eighth Amendment was being debated in 1983. The amendment, which guaranteed the equal right to life of the pregnant woman and the unborn, was, in effect, a constitutional ban on abortion. Mary Robinson describes the treatment of those against the introduction of the amendment as a form of 'political bullying'. As a member of the Seanad at that time, Robinson was against the proposed amendment. 'I did a filibuster on the Eighth Amendment,' she recalls. This was met with 'a certain amount of sniggering and snorting' from some of her colleagues in the Seanad. It has been remarked that at the time the debates on controversial social issues like abortion were so underdeveloped in the political culture 'that neither side was able to relate to the other. And it was a dialogue of the deaf, though not of the mute.'[48]

Looking back at the 1980s, Nora Owen recalls, 'it was a very difficult time in Leinster House. There wasn't as much security [as today], and people seemed to be able to bring visitors into the Dáil, and then just abandon them. You would be walking down a corridor and one of the so-called pro-lifers would stop you and have no compunction about lecturing you about daring to say there's something wrong with the amendment and people shouldn't vote for it.' Owen was one of the Fine Gael TDs who opposed the introduction of the Eighth Amendment in 1983, despite it being introduced by her party leader, Taoiseach Garret FitzGerald. Following lobbying by anti-abortion groups, both Fine Gael and Fianna Fáil had committed to constitutional change. 'I remember when Garret came to the party meeting and said that he had got advice that the wording was going to be fraught with difficulties,' Owen recalls. 'And a number of us said, well then, we shouldn't be going with it.'

Faced with these concerns in his parliamentary party, Owen recalls FitzGerald explaining his predicament: 'He said, "I have given a commitment to this, Charlie Haughey has given a commitment. We will let the people have their say, because if we now say we are not backing an amendment, even though the advice is we don't need it, it will be very difficult for some rural TDs in their constituencies to explain why we are not putting in an amendment to stop abortion."' Looking back on these debates in 1983, Owen admits: 'It was a terribly stupid thing to do. But at the time you kind of had to sit back and say, OK, let the people have their say.'

While Owen was a Fine Gael backbencher during this debate, Gemma Hussey was at cabinet when the challenge in finding a wording that was constitutionally acceptable and would satisfy the anti-abortion groups was debated. 'The discussion about abortion was very political. The actual issue itself wasn't really discussed,' the former Minister for Education recalls. She contrasts the approach in 1983 with today: 'Nobody talked [in 1983] about having had an abortion. I mean, abortion was a real no-no. Nowadays everybody is aware and it's completely different.'

The conservative voices on issues such as contraception, divorce and abortion in the past were both male and female. For example, Hussey and Owen's Fine Gael colleague Alice Glenn was a leading figure in the campaigns to insert the Eighth Amendment into the Irish Constitution in 1983 and to oppose the introduction of divorce in 1986. Her leaflets during the divorce campaign stated that a woman voting for divorce 'is like a turkey voting for Christmas'. Hussey recalls the differing views in Fine Gael under Garret FitzGerald's leadership in the 1980s. 'Garret was in a very difficult position because he was leading a very conservative party,' she explains.

There was a greater homogeneity of viewpoints in Fianna Fáil under the leadership of Charles Haughey, primarily because voices of dissent were given less space. Geoghegan-Quinn had mixed views about the Eighth Amendment but ultimately obeyed the party line. 'All of us did,' she says. 'This was a deal that was done. And the leader of the day said, "This is what we are doing, and this is how it's going to be." Very few people, as I recall it, got up to say anything against it.' As Geoghegan-Quinn states, 'That was the party whip and I obeyed the party whip.' She also explains the pressure on TDs: 'Abortion is always a difficult issue [...] if I was in politics [today], I would be immediately set on by groups as being an abortionist, [being] pro-abortion.'

There was more support in Fianna Fáil for the 1986 divorce referendum. While officially neutral, the party effectively campaigned to see the proposal defeated. Fianna Fáil subsequently supported the second referendum on divorce in 1995, which was accepted. Síle de Valera was always in favour of divorce but opted not to challenge her party's position in the first poll. Like Geoghegan-Quinn, she explains the prevailing attitude of those who may have disagreed with the party's stance: 'The party line is accepted. Like any other issue, you either toe the party line or you don't.' In the second referendum, she publicly stated her support for divorce.

The passage of time and changing social attitudes has seen the approach of the bigger political parties on such issues evolve. For example, Fianna Fáil members were given a free vote in 2013 on the Protection of Life during Pregnancy Bill. Fine Gael, on the other hand, imposed a party whip, and the five TDs and two senators who failed to obey it during the vote on this legislation left the party soon afterwards. In 2018, both Fine Gael and Fianna Fáil adopted a free vote policy on the referendum on the Eighth Amendment. The majority of female TDs in the Dáil chamber favoured removing the amendment, although this was not the case in Fianna Fáil.

An analysis of the 2001 Dáil debate on removing the threat of suicide as a legal ground for abortion showed that female politicians adopted a more liberal position on abortion than their male counterparts. The researchers suggest that this is evidence that gender plays a role in such highly sensitive policy issues.[49] But in the past, it was perhaps more apparent that female TDs, as demonstrated by the stance of Alice Glenn and others, were not a homogenous group. Mary Coughlan, for example, was one of the Fianna Fáil politicians who supported the proposal to remove suicide as a ground for abortion in a 2002 referendum on the issue. 'People have changed within the parliamentary parties, all of the parliamentary parties,' Coughlan observes. 'I suppose I would have been conservative but not intolerant,' she admits. 'My constituency would have been quite conservative. And then I used to get lambasted by people, because I didn't stand up and fly the flag, and tie my bra to the flipping front door of the Dáil, you know. That annoyed me.'

Back then, Coughlan also recalls being confronted with 'the fire and brimstone and our Lord is going to burn us all in hell' as the differing viewpoints contested their respective positions: 'I just hated the polarisation of the views. The middle ground was fine. It's the polarised views that used to drive me crazy. Yet so many people on both sides were intolerant of another perspective. People used to go over the top and that used to drive me nuts.'

※ ※ ※

In 1993, there was another significant and historical change – homosexual acts between consenting men were decriminalised. Moves to change the laws in this area, which dated back to 1861, had been proposed in the Programme for Government agreed by Fianna Fáil and Labour in 1992. Máire Geoghegan-Quinn, who was appointed Minister for Justice in the Albert Reynolds-led coalition, had responsibility for progressing the legislation. There was concern in some Labour circles about the commitment of their larger coalition partners to initiate reform and, in particular, the interest of the new Minister for Justice in progressing the promise.

Geoghegan-Quinn recalls being told of a meeting of Labour politicians at which one representative 'stood up and said, "Lads, we are fucked"'. He was referring to the perceived conservatism of the new Minister for Justice: 'He figured that I was the typical Fianna Fáiler who was right wing on all of these issues and that nothing would happen.' When Geoghegan-Quinn met officials in her new department, they provided a list of proposed legislation with decriminalisation at the very end. The Galway West TD had other ideas.

A Trinity College lecturer, David Norris, had challenged Ireland's policy in Europe. His legal campaign against the criminalisation of homosexuality started in 1977 and was rejected in both the High Court and the Supreme Court before, with the assistance of Mary Robinson, moving to the European Court of Human Rights. The European Court ultimately found that the Irish legal position, dating from the Victorian era, contravened the European Convention on Human Rights. 'I said [to the officials] this is going to come back again. We have to face it head on. Let's do it now,' Geoghegan-Quinn says.

When she brought the draft legislation to the Fianna Fáil parliamentary party, Taoiseach Albert Reynolds said, 'Máire, don't be surprised now and don't be upset if you have a couple of people that will get up and really go to town on this legislation.' She says Reynolds was very supportive: 'Just remember, I'm the leader of the party, I'm backing you 100 per cent.' He need not have been so concerned. Geoghegan-Quinn's proposal met with little resistance. 'Certainly, if anybody had told me when I became Minister for Justice that a piece of legislation that would go through the parliamentary party with virtually just a whimper was the decriminalisation, I wouldn't have believed it.' She says there was subsequently 'a bit of debate' at cabinet but that ultimately there was full support for decriminalisation.

The political tongues of opposition were, however, loosened when the legislation was proceeding through the Oireachtas. Nora Owen recalls what she labels 'gutter speeches' by several politicians. 'My memory of the debate about homosexuals is that the most sympathetic and sensitive speeches were by the women deputies,' she says. Joan Burton was first elected as a Labour TD in the 1992 general election. She also remembers some politicians 'ranting about homosexuality' and a fear in Labour circles that 'widespread revolts' in both Fianna Fáil and Fine Gael would see the legislation defeated. Another new Dáil deputy in 1992, Frances Fitzgerald of Fine Gael, saw the legislation as the start of 'an opening-up period' in Irish society.

The year before homosexuality was decriminalised, President Mary Robinson invited Lesbians Operating Together to Áras an Uachtaráin. The umbrella group had been established in 1991. But none of the representatives who attended released their names to the press.[50] Twenty years later, Katherine Zappone was appointed to the Seanad in 2011 as an Independent and became the first openly lesbian politician in Leinster House. In 2016, she became the first openly lesbian minister to serve in cabinet. When she was first elected to the Seanad, it was important for Zappone to address her sexuality in the chamber, which made some colleagues 'uncomfortable', but she says they got used to her status as a married lesbian. In 2003 Zappone had married fellow academic Ann Louise Gilligan in Canada. Three years later they brought legal proceedings against Revenue for refusing to recognise them as a married couple for tax allowances. Their case was rejected by the High Court.[51] This question would ultimately be resolved in the ballot box and away from the courts. In 2015, more than two decades after decriminalisation legislation was passed into law, the Irish people were asked to vote on permitting same-sex marriage. All political parties supported the referendum. Jan O'Sullivan served as a minister in the Fine Gael–Labour government that proposed the referendum in 2015: 'I think some people who were quite conservative were OK with it, because they never saw it as even possibly affecting them. And in other cases, obviously there was a family member or someone people knew who needed same-sex marriage. So it was a positive, joyful kind of issue.'

The McAleese family fell into the latter category and during the campaign the former president actively campaigned for the referendum to be passed. Mary McAleese spoke about her son, Justin, who she said was born into a society where gay people were denied full citizenship under the Constitution. A Yes vote, she argued at the time, 'costs us nothing. A No vote costs our gay children everything.'[52]

Another former president was monitoring events on the day of the result. 'I have never been prouder of Ireland,' Mary Robinson says. She was in China when the result was declared: 'I had many people coming up, including Chinese, to me and saying, that is a wonderful thing that's happened in your country. And I was very proud of the Irish who came back to vote, sometimes at their own expense. I thought that was incredible.'

The women who have served in senior office since 1979 have been front-seat witnesses to the social changes that have transformed the country. But as the political debates raged, Gemma Hussey believes 'there was a kind of a fear of women [as] divorce, contraception and abortion were all lumped into the same thing'. She points to the influential role of the Catholic Church in helping to defeat proposals like the 1986 divorce referendum: 'I always felt one of the Catholic Church's problems is that they are all so terrified of women, and terrified of women's bodies. They are terrified of their own vulnerability towards women.'

'The Catholic Church still had a huge hold on people,' Nora Owen says of the Ireland that existed in the 1980s. But that clerical hold was diminishing, she thinks. Increasing secularisation augmented by the first abuse scandals in the 1990s combined to lessen the moral authority of the Catholic Church. At a meeting in 1982, in a hotel in Co. Wexford to discuss the setting up of a family planning centre, Father Seán Fortune criticised two Fine Gael TDs who were present in support of the meeting.[53] Fortune later faced multiple charges of child sex abuse.

As a government minister in the 1990s, Labour's Niamh Bhreathnach witnessed this dramatic shift in influence: 'The role of the Catholic Church has diminished so much [that] there is now a new space to hear more voices. And they were the least voices you heard [previously] – women's voices.' People are now no longer willing to be dictated to about what they should think, Jan O'Sullivan says: 'It's kind of chicken and egg. I think the Catholic Church is in a weaker position because people have decided that they want to make their own decisions. And then because the Catholic Church is in a weaker position, then they don't have the same influence that they had before.'

Mary McAleese believes the Catholic Church 'is in end-stage terminal illness, even though it is growing worldwide in terms of numbers. But those numbers are bogus, because they are predicated upon the child who is born, who is baptised at two weeks and their baptism now makes them, according to canon law, a member of the church with all the rights and obligations. That process, of its very nature, is utterly bogus.' As the former president says: 'We are now dealing with the single most educated cohort of Irish people in the history of Ireland. We got access to free second-level education … [which] really began to kick in, in the 1970s. And because that massified, so too in turn did third-level education. Now we have people who are equipped with intellectual skills and analytical skills bar none. You can't plámás them anymore with shibboleths.'

In the 2018 referendum to remove the Eighth Amendment, one in ten of those surveyed in the RTÉ exit poll cited religious views as an influencing factor in how they voted. The Fine Gael minister Josepha Madigan, who was co-ordinator of her party's campaign to repeal the amendment, believes: 'There's definitely been a shift. I think Irish society is ready to extricate itself from that institutional mindset, where we all just do what we are told and we all follow a certain protocol just because we are told to do it. And that's probably a good thing.' Part of these shifts in public opinion has created a society where there is a much greater openness and space to discuss contentious social and moral issues, according to Síle de Valera: 'Before, we had a cloudy view of what the issues were. Nobody would talk about a case study or give their personal view. But now they are talked openly, thankfully.'

The idea of politicians telling personal stories and naming members of the public to emphasise their arguments was previously unacceptable, Mary Hanafin says. The former Fianna Fáil minister claims many of her colleagues 'would have knocked you down' if you had imparted a personal experience in a Dáil speech. This reticence, she believes, was partly due to the traditional formality of Dáil proceedings. But Hanafin acknowledges the role of Oireachtas committees in discussing social issues, which in turn has led to the environment being 'more collegial and lends itself to greater insights, greater debate, greater sharing of experiences'. Heather Humphreys, who was first elected in 2011, believes male politicians are also now 'more comfortable giving their personal stories', largely because such policies are no longer considered as separate silos designated as either male or female issues.

Mary Coughlan experienced an example of this change as a government minister when the BreastCheck programme was discussed at cabinet. 'That came up as a health issue as opposed to a women's issue,' Coughlan explains. Her male ministerial colleagues were under as much pressure to deliver the programme as the women at cabinet. 'The men that are elected now are different to the people that were before them,' she says, explaining that many ministers today are young men with young families.

Former Tánaiste Joan Burton has also seen changes in how sensitive social issues are discussed in the Oireachtas: 'There is definitely a very big difference. It's much more civilised. And it is much more acknowledging that people have their right to their views, and they have a right to have those views respected. That has been a very strong positive.' Another former Tánaiste, the first woman to hold the title, Mary Harney believes the presence of more female representatives in Leinster House has helped change the nature of conversations in political life. However, she also acknowledges that 'society has changed, and the political system is somewhat behind society in that regard'.

Katherine Zappone, a former chief executive of the National Women's Council, acknowledges the role played by women's groups. Other female politicians highlight the influence of Ireland's membership of the European Union in driving much of social change over the last half-century. 'You know, just being part of that wider Europe culturally opened us up,' Mary Robinson argues. During her political career, Síle de Valera served in the European Parliament from 1979 to 1984. She saw first-hand the European influence on Ireland: 'The European Parliament at that stage would have been very much ahead of what was happening in Ireland in terms of women's equality. Their policies [on] paternity leave, maternity leave, equal rights for women within the working place were comparatively new to us. And certainly, new in a legislative sense, in the way they discussed it.' De Valera highlights the value in more women entering politics and being in a position to influence such decisions. She says there has been 'more of an acceptance of the right of women in all spheres of life. And that kind of approach to equality began to influence the work in the Dáil.'

The profile of the women taking part in national politics has also evolved. In the 1970s, Mary Robinson and Gemma Hussey, and later in the 1980s and 1990s, Mary McAleese, Niamh Bhreathnach, Frances Fitzgerald and Joan Burton emerged onto the stage without the aid of political family connections. Indeed, twelve of the nineteen women who have served as senior ministers are not related to a previous representative in Leinster House. Of those twelve, two had a parent who was politically involved – in the case of Regina Doherty, her mother was an unsuccessful local election candidate for Fine Gael, while Josepha Madigan's father was a local councillor first for Fianna Fáil and then as an Independent.

After the 2011 general election, for the first time in the history of the state, no female TDs were related to a former TD. In 2016, just two women had links to a previous office-holder.[54] This is in sharp contrast to the DNA of the female TDs who served between 1922 and 1977. During this period, just 24 women were elected to the Dáil, and 80 per cent were related to a former male TD.[55] While the women born into political dynasties acknowledge the electoral weight of their surnames, several were challenged about their credentials, not only in terms of their gender, but also, in the case of daughters running for office, their youth.

Irrespective of their political backgrounds, on the campaign trail in the 1970s and 1980s, many women came face-to-face with social judgements on their decision to run for office and work outside the home. In a reply to a questionnaire in 1977, one Fianna Fáil TD, Tim O'Connor, noted that, 'in my own county the women are doing a great job of work in keeping their homes going and bringing up families. This, I think, is just what Almighty God intended them to do.'[56] Times may have changed since O'Connor's declaration in 1977 but Jan O'Sullivan holds the view that there is still a 'residual thing that really your first responsibility is to be at home with your kids'. The former Labour minister believes that there is still a perception among some people that the cut and thrust of politics is for 'somebody whose children are reared or who doesn't have children'.

❧ ❧ ❧

The vast majority of women who have served in cabinet believe it was tougher for them to break into national politics because those already serving in office had a clear advantage and those incumbents have been, historically, male. Their views are supported by an analysis of first-preference votes in the 2016 general election.[57] This analysis showed that female candidates won over a half a million first-preference votes (25 per cent of the total votes cast) in this election for the first time. This figure represents an increase of almost 200,000 votes on the number of first preferences won by female candidates in the 2011 election and is largely attributed to the higher number of women running for election due to gender quotas.

However, despite the increased first-preference votes, male candidates won, on average, 830 more votes than female candidates. The 2016 picture stands in contrast to 2011 where women candidates received slightly more first-preference votes on average than men. The researchers point to incumbency as a likely factor in 2016. Just under 5 per cent of all candidates were female incumbents, compared to 22 per cent of candidates who were male incumbents. A review of the vote share showed incumbents received an average vote of 7,249 compared to 2,665 for non-incumbents.

Others point to a mindset within political parties. Máire Geoghegan-Quinn is of the view that women have tended to be 'the soft target' when parties showed preference between male and female candidates: 'Almost always the target will become the woman [...] like, God we could never sacrifice so-and-so's seat because he's so vital and so important.'

Most of the female ministers believe the introduction of gender quotas and the record level of female representation in 2016 marks the beginning of significant change in our national parliament. There is a growing acceptance inside and outside

Leinster House that the gender balance in Irish politics needs to be addressed. The introduction of gender quotas forced the political parties to act. The women who have served in cabinet remember, however, that there have been false dawns in the past. 'When Mary Robinson was elected, there was a great impetus to push hard to get more women,' Mary Coughlan says. 'Remember, we got the greatest number of women elected at the time. And that was good. But it's terrible to think that we are still talking about it.'

Robinson is equally disappointed: 'We are not seeing an encouragement of women to come forward. I think the party system isn't naturally one that women will find very comfortable.' Frances Fitzgerald agrees: 'You have to be very proactive to get women to engage in politics'. She points out that there are 'still more ambitious young men coming through than young ambitious women as it happens in party politics'. Mary Hanafin has also noticed this trend: 'We are finding it very hard to get young women in. It's mostly young men now who are joining.' However, she believes 'there's now an expectation that every party in every constituency will be running women. It's just now taken as a given.'

A lot of work remains to be done, according to Fine Gael's Mary Mitchell O'Connor, to get 'that critical mass of women within Dáil Éireann'. But Mary McAleese is optimistic about the future and of more women attaining senior political positions: 'We are beginning to throw off the shackles regarding women as only suited to certain kinds of areas. And partly it is because we are now invading those areas that we didn't invade before. Whenever I was in law school, there were almost fifty in my class, of whom ten were women. If I went into a law school now, and there were fifty in the class, you could be sure that forty will be women and ten will be men.'

Many in the political system hope that there will be a domino effect – that the election of more female TDs will ultimately lead to the appointment of more women to cabinet positions. But that does not explain or excuse the meagre number of women who have attained senior ministerial office. The paltry number appointed to cabinet positions over almost 100 years is an indictment of the political system and political leadership since the foundation of the state. If more women are elected to the Dáil following the introduction of the gender-quota system, their promotional prospects depend on the political will of the Taoiseach of the day or the other party leader in a coalition government. There is also a queue for political advancement with fierce competition for positions. There are signs that gender will be a strong consideration in future appointments, but it remains to be seen if it will have the same weight as geography and length of service.

❧ ❧ ❧

On the pages of *Madam Politician*, the stories of the seventeen surviving women who sat around the cabinet table and the two former presidents who were elected head of state have come to life. These women are trailblazers, confronting long-standing prejudices and the barriers that limited women's participation in all levels of Irish politics. The era of a single woman at the cabinet table in an overwhelmingly male-dominated team is long gone. In fact, the idea that just two or even three women would sit at the table now seems to belong to a different time. The 2018 cabinet appointments in Spain are proof that it is not unrealistic to have equality between men and women in political life, and even for women to hold a majority of positions in government. Many of the Irish female ministers believe equality of numbers, based on ability and experience, brings an additional dynamic to policy-making and ultimately leads to better decisions in the public interest.

In their successes and triumphs, their errors and mistakes, the nineteen women who have served as senior ministers have shown they are little different than their male counterparts. However, as we approach the third decade of the 21st century, female politicians face specific challenges, which are different to their male colleagues. There is the relentless focus on their appearance by the media and voters along with various levels of sexism as identified by the #metoo movement in all areas of society.

The years to come will test the progress of women in Irish political life. The verdict will be based on a variety of outcomes – will the number of women serving as senior ministers have increased significantly? If so, will these changes be sustained? Will the political hue of the women in senior office have broadened? Will Irish women finally have broken the remaining glass ceilings in political life? Perhaps progress will be most evident when such commentary becomes redundant and it is as normal for large numbers of women – as it is for men – to attain senior office without sensational headlines or extensive commentary about their appointments.

During the Dublin Theatre Festival in 2015, Mary Robinson attended a performance of *The Train*, a play based on the stories of the women who travelled to Belfast in 1971 to buy contraceptives, which were banned in the Republic at the time. Robinson was accompanied to the play by her niece Rebecca. The former president was struck by her niece's surprise that having access to contraception was ever an issue for women in Ireland: 'My niece, who is a bright intelligent woman, couldn't believe that this had happened. She could not believe that this had been the case so recently. In other words, her complete unawareness of what it had been like.' For Robinson, this in itself, was 'an example of success'. The task now is to replicate this type of reaction in terms of women's role in Irish political life and specifically at the cabinet table. When it is no longer necessary to discuss the number of women attaining senior political office, real change will have taken place.

The journey of the women who climbed the political ladder with mettle and determination and who overcame so many practical challenges and closed mind-sets should never be forgotten. The journey started in 1919, a year after Irish women were first allowed to vote, albeit in limited circumstances. The journey started with Countess Constance Markievicz, who later said in a Dáil debate on the role of women in society:

> *This question of votes for women, with the bigger thing, freedom for women and the opening up of the professions to women, has been one of the things that I have worked for and given my influence and time to procuring all my life whenever I got an opportunity. I have worked in Ireland, I have even worked in England to help the women obtain their freedom. I would work for it anywhere, as one of the crying wrongs of the world, that women, because of their sex, should be debarred from any position or any right that their brains entitle them a right to hold.*[58]

Appendix:
Female Presidents
and Ministers

Presidents

1. **Mary Robinson** was elected President of Ireland in 1990. She
    succeeded six men who had previously held the position of
    head of state. She was a member of Seanad Éireann from 1969
    to 1989. During this time, she gained national recognition as
    a leading human rights lawyer and Reid Professor of Criminal
    Law at Trinity College, Dublin. She was an unsuccessful
    Labour candidate in the 1977 and 1981 general elections
    but did serve a term as an elected member of Dublin City
    Council (1979–83). She opted not to seek a second term as
    president in 1997. Robinson served as United Nations High
    Commissioner for Human Rights between 1997 and 2002.
    She currently leads the Mary Robinson Foundation – Climate
    Justice.

2. **Mary McAleese** was elected President of Ireland in 1997.
    She secured a second seven-year term without an election in
    2004. She was the first person born in Northern Ireland to be
    elected head of state in the Republic of Ireland. Previously,
    she was pro-vice-chancellor of Queen's University in Belfast.
    She also worked as a current affairs broadcaster with RTÉ and
    as an academic lawyer, succeeding Mary Robinson as Reid

Professor at Trinity College, Dublin. She was a member of the Catholic Church's delegation to the New Ireland Forum in 1984. She was an unsuccessful Fianna Fáil candidate in the 1987 general election. Since leaving the presidency, Mary McAleese has campaigned for same-sex marriage and has been a leading advocate for the reform of the Catholic Church.

Ministers

1. **Countess Constance Markievicz** was the first Irish woman ever to hold a cabinet position when she became Minister for Labour in 1919. Born Constance Georgine Gore-Booth, she was also the first woman elected to the House of Commons in 1918, although along with the other Sinn Féin MPs, she did not take her seat at Westminster. Markievicz fought in the 1916 Easter Rising and was sentenced to death for her involvement; this was later commuted to life in prison. She was one of the founding members of Fianna Fáil in 1926. Markievicz died in 1927.

2. **Máire Geoghegan-Quinn** was first elected to the Dáil for Fianna Fáil in Galway West in 1975, following the death of her father, Johnny Geoghegan. She became the country's second female cabinet minister in 1979, and the first since the foundation of the state in 1922, when she was appointed Minister for the Gaeltacht. In 1992, she was appointed Minister for Tourism, Transport and Communications. She was the first female Minister for Justice (1993–94) and in 1994 also briefly had responsibility for the Department of Equality and Law Reform. Geoghegan-Quinn retired from national politics at the 1997 general election.

3. **Eileen Desmond** was first elected to the Dáil in the Cork Mid constituency in 1965, following the death of her husband,

Dan, who was a Labour TD. During the 1981–82 Fine Gael–Labour coalition, she was appointed Minister for Health and Social Welfare. She also served in the Seanad (1969–1973) and the European Parliament (1979–1984). She retired from national politics at the 1987 general election. Desmond died in 2005.

4. **Gemma Hussey** was first elected a TD in February 1982 for Fine Gael in Wicklow. She was the first woman appointed as Minister for Education in December 1982. In a cabinet reshuffle in February 1986, she was appointed Minister for Social Welfare. She was briefly Minister for Labour in 1987 after Labour left the Fine Gael-led coalition government. Prior to her service in the Dáil, Hussey had been a senator between 1977, when she was elected as an Independent to the NUI panel, and 1982. Hussey retired from national politics in 1989.

5. **Mary O'Rourke** was first elected to Dáil Éireann in November 1982 for Longford–Westmeath. Several family members have also been Fianna Fáil TDs, including her father Paddy Lenihan (1965–70). Her brother Brian Lenihan and two of his sons held ministerial positions in various Fianna Fáil-led governments. Her political career in Leinster House included appointments as Minister for Education (1987–1991), Minister for Health (1991–1992) and Minister for Public Enterprise (1997–2002). She was deputy leader of Fianna Fáil from 1994 to 2002, the first woman to hold this position. O'Rourke retired from national politics after the 2011 general election.

6. **Niamh Bhreathnach** was elected as a Labour TD for Dún Laoghaire in November 1992. She became a cabinet minister following her election when she was appointed Minister for Education in the Fianna Fáil–Labour coalition in January

1993. When the government collapsed, she was re-appointed to the same portfolio in the subsequent Rainbow Coalition made up of Fine Gael, Labour and Democratic Left (1994–97). She lost her Dáil seat in 1997 and was an unsuccessful candidate five years later. Bhreathnach retired from national politics after the 2002 general election.

7. **Nora Owen** was first elected to the Dáil in 1981 as a Fine Gael TD for Dublin North. A grand-niece of Michael Collins, she was appointed deputy leader of Fine Gael in 1993, becoming the first woman to hold the position. When the Rainbow Coalition was formed in 1994, she was appointed Minister for Justice. Owen retired from national politics after the 2002 general election.

8. **Mary Harney** was first elected to the Dáil in 1981 for Fianna Fáil in Dublin South-West. She was one of the founding members of the Progressive Democrats. She was elected Progressive Democrats leader in 1993, and in doing so became the first woman to lead an Irish political party in the Dáil. She held the position until 2006. She led her party into a coalition government with Fianna Fáil in 1997, when she became the first woman to be appointed Tánaiste. Over the following fourteen years she served as Minister for Enterprise, Trade and Employment (1997–2004) and Minister for Health and Children (2004–11). Mary Harney retired from national politics at the 2011 general election, at which point she was the longest-serving female TD in the history of the Irish state.

9. **Síle de Valera** first won a Dáil seat for Fianna Fáil in 1977 in the Dublin County Mid constituency and later represented the Clare constituency. She is a granddaughter of Éamon de Valera, Fianna Fáil's first leader and a former Taoiseach and

president. She was appointed Minister for the Arts, Heritage, Gaeltacht and the Islands in 1997 but lost her cabinet position in 2002. De Valera retired from national politics at the 2007 general election.

10. **Mary Coughlan** was first elected a TD in 1987 for Donegal South-West at the age of 21. She succeeded her father, Cathal, and uncle, Clement, who had both served as Fianna Fáil TDs for the same constituency. She was first appointed to cabinet as Minister for Social and Family Affairs (2002–04) and later was the first woman to serve as Minister for Agriculture (2004–08). She was also Minister for Enterprise, Trade and Employment (2008–10), Minister for Education and Skills (2010–11) and briefly Minister for Health and Children in early 2011. She was deputy leader of Fianna Fáil from 2008 to 2011, during which time she was also Tánaiste. Coughlan retired from national politics after the 2011 general election.

11. **Mary Hanafin** was first elected to the Dáil in 1997 in Dún Laoghaire. Her father, Des Hanafin, was a senator, as was her brother John. She served as Minister for Education and Science (2004–08), Minister for Social and Family Affairs (2008–10) and Minister for Tourism, Culture and Sport (2010–11). She was briefly Minister for Enterprise, Trade and Innovation in early 2011. She was deputy leader of Fianna Fáil for two months at the start of 2011. Hanafin lost her Dáil seat in the 2011 general election and was again unsuccessful in 2016.

12. **Joan Burton** was first elected to the Dáil for Labour in Dublin West in 1992. She was elected deputy leader of her party in 2007. When the Fine Gael–Labour coalition was formed in 2011 she was appointed Minister for Social Protection. She succeeded Eamon Gilmore as Labour leader in 2014 and became the first woman to hold that position. She was

subsequently appointed Tánaiste. Joan Burton held her seat at the 2016 general election.

13. **Frances Fitzgerald** was first elected to the Dáil for Fine Gael in Dublin South-East in 1992 and later won a seat in the Dublin Mid-West constituency. She served as Minister for Children and Youth Affairs (2011–14), Minister for Justice and Equality (2014–17) and Minister for Business, Enterprise and Innovation (2017). She was appointed Tánaiste in 2016, becoming the second Fine Gael politician to hold the position and the first woman from her party. Fitzgerald held her seat at the 2016 general election, but resigned from cabinet in November 2017 over a garda whistle-blower controversy.

14. **Jan O'Sullivan** was first elected in a Dáil by-election in Limerick East in 1998 following the death of her long-time colleague, Jim Kemmy. Along with Kemmy, she joined Labour in 1990 following a merger with their Democratic Socialist Party. She was appointed Minister for Education and Skills in July 2014 following a cabinet reshuffle when Joan Burton replaced Eamon Gilmore as Labour leader. O'Sullivan held her seat at the 2016 general election.

15. **Heather Humphreys** was first elected to the Dáil in 2011 in Cavan–Monaghan for Fine Gael. She has served as Minister for Arts, Heritage and the Gaeltacht (2014–16), Minister for Arts, Heritage, Regional, Rural and Gaeltacht Affairs (2016–17), Minister for Culture, Heritage and the Gaeltacht (2017) and since November 2017 as Minister for Business, Enterprise and Innovation.

16. **Mary Mitchell O'Connor** was first elected to the Dáil in 2011 for Fine Gael in Dún Laoghaire. She was appointed to the cabinet in the Fine Gael–Independent minority government in May 2016 and served as Minister for Jobs, Enterprise and Innovation until June 2017.

17. **Katherine Zappone** was first elected as an Independent TD in Dublin South-West in the 2016 general election. She was appointed as an Independent minister in the Fine Gael-led minority coalition in May 2016. She currently serves as Minister for Children and Youth Affairs. She is one of only six TDs to be appointed to cabinet after being first elected to the Dáil.

18. **Regina Doherty** was first elected to the Dáil in 2011 for Fine Gael in the Meath East constituency. She was appointed Minister for Employment Affairs and Social Protection in June 2017 following the election of Leo Varadkar as Taoiseach.

19. **Josepha Madigan** was first elected to the Dáil in 2016 in the Dublin–Rathdown constituency for Fine Gael. She became a senior cabinet minister in November 2017 when she was appointed Minister for Culture, Heritage and the Gaeltacht.

REFERENCES

Ahern, Bertie, with Richard Aldous, *The Autobiography* (Hutchinson, 2009).

Andrews, David, *Kingstown Republican: A Memoir,* (New Island, 2007).

Arnold, Bruce, *Haughey: His Life and Unlucky Deeds,* (HarperCollins, 1994).

Baumann, Markus, Debus, Marc and Müller, Jochen, 'Convictions and Signals in Parliamentary Speeches: Dáil Éireann Debates on Abortion in 2001 and 2013', *Irish Political Studies* (30:2), 199–219.

Boyle, Dan, *Without Power or Glory: The Greens in Government* (New Island, 2012).

Buckley, Fiona, 'Women and Politics in Ireland: The Road to Sex Quotas', *Irish Political Studies* (28:3), 341–359.

Buckley, Fiona, Galligan, Yvonne and McGing, Claire, 'Women and the Election: Assessing the Impact of Gender Quotas', in Michael Gallagher and Michael Marsh (eds) *How Ireland Voted 2016: The Election that Nobody Won* (Palgrave Macmillan, 2016).

Claffey, Úna, *The Women Who Won: Women of the 27th Dáil* (Attic Press, 1993).

Clinton, Hillary Rodham, *What Happened* (Simon & Schuster, 2017)

Collins, Stephen, *Breaking the Mould: How the PDs Changed Irish Politics* (Gill and Macmillan, 2005).

Collins, Stephen, *The Power Game: Fianna Fáil since Lemass* (O'Brien Press, 2000).

Collins, Stephen, *Spring and the Labour Story* (O'Brien Press, 1993).

Connolly, Eileen, 'Parliaments as Gendered Institutions: The Irish Oireachtas', *Irish Political Studies* (28:3), 360–379.

Desmond, Barry, *Finally and in Conclusion: A Political Memoir* (New Island, 2000).

Duignan, Seán, *One Spin on the Merry-Go-Round* (Blackwater Press, 1995).

Ferriter, Diarmaid, *Occasions of Sin, Sex and Society in Modern Ireland* (Profile Books, 2009).

Finlay, Fergus, *Snakes and Ladders* (New Island, 1998).

FitzGerald, Garret, *An Autobiography* (Macmillan, 1991).

Foster, R.F., *Luck and the Irish: A Brief History of Change, 1970–2000* (Penguin, 2008).

Galligan, Yvonne, 'Activist Presidents and Gender Politics, 1990–2011', in John Coakley and Kevin Rafter (eds), *The Irish Presidency: Power, Ceremony and Politics* (Irish Academic Press, 2014).

Galligan, Yvonne and Buckley, Fiona, 'Women in Politics', in John Coakley and Michael Gallagher (eds) *Politics in the Republic of Ireland, Sixth Edition* (Routledge, 2018).

Gilligan, Ann Louise and Zappone, Katherine, *Our Lives Out Loud: In Pursuit of Justice and Equality*, (O'Brien Press, 2008).

Gilmore, Eamon, *Inside the Room: The Untold Story of Ireland's Crisis Government*, (Merrion, 2016).

Haverty, Anne, *Constance Markievicz: Irish Revolutionary* (Lilliput, 2016).

Hussey, Gemma, *At the Cutting Edge: Cabinet Diaries 1982–1987*, (Gill and Macmillan, 1990).

Joyce, Joe and Murtagh, Peter, *The Boss: Charles J. Haughey in Government* (Poolbeg, 1983).

Kavanagh, Ray, *Spring, Summer and Fall: The Rise and Fall of the Labour Party, 1986–1999* (Blackwater, 2001).

Leahy, Pat, *Showtime: The Inside Story of Fianna Fáil in Power* (Penguin, 2009).

Leahy, Pat, *The Price of Power: Inside Ireland's Crisis Coalition* (Penguin, 2013).

Lee, J.J., *Ireland 1912–1988: Politics and Society* (Cambridge University Press, 1989).

Lee, John and McConnell, Daniel, *Hell at the Gates: The Inside of Ireland's Financial Downfall* (Mercier, 2016).

MacMánais, Ray, *The Road from Ardoyne: The Making of a President* (Brandon, 2004).

McAuliffe, Mary and Gillis, Liz, *Richmond Barracks 1916: We Were There – 77 Women of the Easter Rising* (Dublin City Council, 2016).

McCarthy, Justine, *Mary McAleese: The Outsider* (Blackwater, 1999).

McElroy, Gail and Marsh, Michael, 'Electing Women to the Dáil: Gender Cues and the Irish Voter', *Irish Political Studies* (26:4), 521–534.

McGing, Claire, 'The Single Transferable Vote and Women's Representation in Ireland', *Irish Political Studies* (28:3), 322–340.

McGing, Claire and White, Timothy, 'Gender and Electoral Representation in Ireland', *Études Irlandaises* (37:2), pp. 33–48.

O'Brien, Anne, 'It's a Man's World: A Qualitative Study of the (Non) Mediation of Women and Politics on *Prime Time* During the 2011 General Election', *Irish Political Studies* (29:4), 505–521.

O'Byrnes, Stephen, *Hiding Behind a Face: Fine Gael Under FitzGerald* (Gill and Macmillan, 1986).

O'Leary, Olivia and Burke, Helen, *Mary Robinson: The Authorised Biography* (Hodder and Stoughton, 1998).

O'Malley, Desmond, *Conduct Unbecoming: A Memoir* (Gill and Macmillan, 2014).

O'Malley, Eoin, 'Ministerial Selection in Ireland: Limited Choice in a Political Village', *Irish Political Studies* (21:3), 319–336.

O'Rourke, Mary, *Just Mary: A Memoir* (Gill and Macmillan, 2012).

Quinn, Ruairi, *Straight Left: A Journey in Politics* (Hodder Headline, 2005).

Rafter, Kevin, *Fine Gael: Party at the Crossroads* (New Island, 2009).

Reynolds, Albert, *My Autobiography* (Transworld Ireland, 2009).

Robinson, Mary, *Everybody Matters: A Memoir* (Hodder and Stoughton, 2012).

Ward, Margaret, *In Their Own Voice: Women and Irish Nationalism* (Attic, 1995).

Yates, Ivan, *Full On: A Memoir,* (Hachette Ireland, 2014).

NOTES

1   Anne Haverty, *Constance Markievicz: Irish Revolutionary* (Lilliput, 2016), p.96.

2   Yvonne Galligan and Fiona Buckley, 'Women in Politics', in John Coakley and Michael Gallagher (eds) *Politics in the Republic of Ireland, Sixth Edition* (Routledge, 2018), p.222.

3   Ibid., p.220.

4   Greg Harkin, '"A woman as Taoiseach, we will have to wait and see": 14 female ministers gather to celebrate Countess Markievicz', *Irish Independent*, 16 July 2016.

5   Galligan and Buckley, p.217.

6   RTÉ, 'Women in Irish Society' (http://www.rte.ie/archives/exhibitions/1666-women-and-society/).

7   Galligan and Buckley, p.219.

8   Hillary Rodham Clinton, *What Happened* (Simon & Schuster, 2017), p.119.

9   Eoin O'Malley, 'Ministerial Selection in Ireland: Limited Choice in a Political Village', *Irish Political Studies* (21:3), p.333–34.

10   Galligan and Buckley, p.224.

11   Úna Claffey, *The Women Who Won* (Attic Press, 1993), p.156.

12   Seán Duignan. *One Spin on the Merry-Go-Round*, (Blackwater, 1995), p.17.

13   Claffey, p.34.

14   Information provided by Oireachtas Library and Research Service, 2017.

15   Gail McElroy and Michael Marsh, 'Electing Women to the Dáil: Gender Cues and the Irish Voter', *Irish Political Studies* (26:4), p. 532.

16   Ibid., p.533.

17   Fiona Buckley, 'Women and Politics in Ireland: The Road to Sex Quotas', *Irish Political Studies* (28:3), p.354.

18   Fiona Buckley, Yvonne Galligan and Claire McGing, 'Women and the Election: Assessing the Impact of Gender Quotas', in Michael Gallagher and Michael Marsh (eds) *How Ireland Voted 2016: The Election that Nobody Won* (Palgrave Macmillan, 2016), p.196.

19 Inter-Parliamentary Union, January 2018 (http://archive.ipu.org/wmn-e/classif.htm).

20 Buckley, Galligan and McGing, p.199.

21 Cormac McQuinn, 'Wide support for gender quotas in local elections', *Irish Independent*, 8 August 2017; 'Call for introduction of gender quotas in local elections', Conor McMorrow, RTÉ.ie, 7 June 2018; '#NowWhatsNext', Women For Election: (www.womenforelection.ie/campaigns/nowwhatsnext/).

22 Claire Annesley, 'How a "concrete floor" could get more women into power', BBC News, 5 June 2018.

23 Ciara Meehan, '1970s Ireland: A Good Place for Women?' (https://ciarameehan.com/2013/05/27/1970s-ireland-a-good-place-for-women/).

24 Leaflet available at Irish Election Literature website: https://irishelectionliterature.com/tag/womens-political-association/.

25 Claire McGing and Timothy J. White, 'Gender and Electoral Representation in Ireland', *Études Irlandaises* (37:2).

26 Information courtesy of Iain McMenamin, Dublin City University.

27 Barry Desmond, *Finally and in Conclusion: A Political Memoir* (New Island, 2000), p.325.

28 Desmond O'Malley, *Conduct Unbecoming: A Memoir* (Gill and Macmillan, 2014), p.186.

29 President Mary Robinson's Acceptance Speech, 9 November 1990 (http://www.president.ie/en/media-library/speeches/president-robinsons-acceptance-speech).

30 Galligan and Buckley, p.220.

31 Yvonne Galligan, 'Activist Presidents and Gender Politics, 1990–2011', in John Coakley, John and Kevin Rafter (eds), *The Irish Presidency: Power, Ceremony and Politics*, (Irish Academic Press, 2014), p.126.

32 Ibid., p.146.

33 Mary Robinson; Inauguration Speech, 3 December 1990.

34 Mary Robinson, *Everybody Matters: A Memoir* (Hodder and Stoughton, 2012), p.173.

35 Galligan, p.141.

36 Robinson. p.167.

37 Mary Minihan, 'Norris regrets any offence caused by "fanny" remark', *The Irish Times*, 17 July 2013.

38   'Vanity Fair sorry for suggesting Hillary Clinton "knit"', BBC News, 28 December 2017.

39   Irish Sun and Irish Mirror, 19 June 1998.

40   Irish Mirror, 19 June 1998.

41   'TD had offered to quit before', The Irish Times, 19 February 2001.

42   'Tom Barry "severely reprimanded" by Fine Gael general secretary', RTÉ News, 17 July 2013.

43   Diarmaid Ferriter, Occasions of Sin, Sex and Society in Modern Ireland (Profile Books, 2009), pp.443–44.

44   Ibid., p.410.

45   J.J. Lee, Ireland 1912–1988: Politics and Society (Cambridge University Press, 1989), p.656.

46   Ferriter, p.407.

47   Ferriter, p.441.

48   Lee, p.655.

49   Markus Baumann, Marc Debus and Jochen Müller, 'Convictions and Signals in Parliamentary Speeches: Dáil Éireann Debates on Abortion in 2001 and 2013', Irish Political Studies (30:2).

50   Ferriter, p.515.

51   'Lesbian couple lose marriage recognition case', RTÉ News, 14 December 2016.

52   'No vote will "cost our children everything" – McAleese', RTÉ News, 19 May 2015.

53   Ferriter, p.472.

54   Buckley, Galligan and McGing, p.199.

55   Galligan and Buckley, p.229.

56   R.F. Foster, Luck and the Irish: A Brief History of Change, 1970–2000 (Penguin, 2008), p.41.

57   Buckley, Galligan and McGing, pp.197–78.

58   Countess Markievicz from Dáil Éireann debate on Irish women and the extension of the franchise, 2 March 1922, in Margaret Ward, In Their Own Voice: Women and Irish Nationalism (Attic Press, 1995), p.135.

INDEX